Trigger Point Therapy

Massagers and Manual Back Massagers to Relieve Pain

(Learn Trigger Point Therapy by Using Body Tools to Apply Pressure to Yourself)

Imogene Collins

Published By **Ryan Princeton**

Imogene Collins

Trigger Point Therapy: Massagers and Manual Back Massagers to Relieve Pain (Learn Trigger Point Therapy by Using Body Tools to Apply Pressure to Yourself)

ISBN 978-1-998769-61-2

Legal & Disclaimer

Table of contents

Chapter 1: Understanding Trigger Point Therapy

Pain lets you know when something is wrong. In fact, it's designed to divert your attention away from other tasks and toward the area where you're experiencing pain. Inevitably, this creates various difficulties, and it can prevent you from enjoying your life and performing your daily activities.

To treat trigger points, you ideally would have a method that eliminates your pain, and then stops it from coming back. This is where self-performed trigger point therapy can play a very beneficial part.

However, understanding trigger point therapy starts with uncovering what went wrong in the first place. Why are you experiencing pain? What is going on beneath the surface?

Trigger points are the most common cause of muscle pain in humans. They can cause pain, stiffness, and disability. Below, we're going to explore what trigger points are in more detail, as well as how to treat your triggers and make them go away.

What Are Trigger Points?

A trigger point is a tiny and sensitive area on a muscle that has gone into spasm, and therefore causes pain.

It is usually the size of your fingernail, and when you press on it, it hurts. Additionally, you might notice pain appearing in nearby structures or muscles.

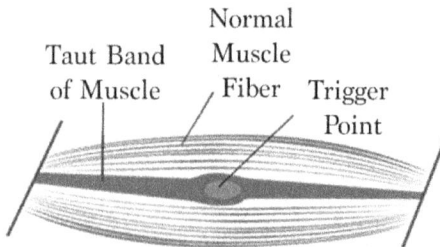

The Trigger Point Complex

Each active trigger point has an area where it causes pain. This is called the pain referral pattern. These patterns were mapped out in the sixties by Doctors Travell and Simons. Where you feel pain will depend on your specific trigger point and its pain referral pattern.

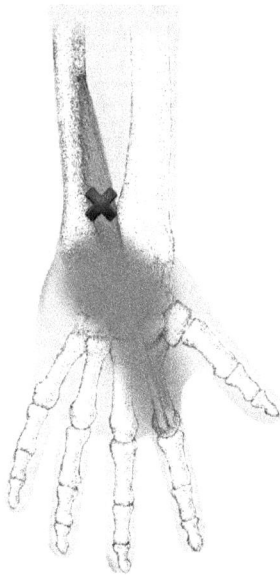

A trigger point (the X) and its pain referral pattern (in red)

Surprisingly, trigger points aren't well recognized or understood by most doctors. They aren't taught in medical school, mostly because it's difficult to subject this type of pain to a double blinded placebo study. This doesn't make them any less real.

(You can see some more recent studies of trigger points here.)

The Science Behind Trigger Points & Trigger Point Therapy

Trigger points are a neuromuscular problem involving the nerves and muscle spindles. Inside each muscle, there are millions of tiny muscle spindles. These muscle spindles are shaped like a spring, wrapped around the muscle fiber, and they have the ability to recoil.

For example, when you stretch your bicep muscle, the spindles also stretch. When you reach a critical point of the stretch, these muscle spindles send signals that you're about to stretch the muscle too far. These messages go to the spinal cord, which then directs your muscle to contract. This protective reflex prevents your muscles and joints from being over extended.

However, these muscle spindles are also at the centre of what goes wrong when a trigger point occurs. For example, if you were to trip and fall, your muscle spindles would send a frantic message to your spinal cord to protect you and contract the necessary muscles.

After this protective phase, the muscle spindles should return to their normal state within a few hours. Trigger points happen when the spindles go into a protective mode and don't return to their normal state.

Instead, they get stuck in this protective mode. When this happens, you experience muscle stiffness and soreness. The stressed muscle has a micro-spasm in it, because the trigger point will not turn off. Left alone, trigger points can persist for weeks or even years, and this creates knock-on ill effects on your muscle health and mobility.

Successful trigger treatment interferes with the reflex loop your body is stuck in. It switches off and resets the muscle spindles. This is how trigger point therapy can help alleviate your muscle pain.

The Two Types of Trigger Points

Before we dive into how to perform trigger point therapy, it's important to differentiate between the two types of trigger points. The two types of trigger points are active triggers and latent triggers.

Active triggers are when the spot is really sore and tender to touch. When you press on it, there's pain in the trigger point, and also in the pain referral pathway of that trigger. You may also experience muscle spasm and tightness.

Latent triggers are when the spot is no longer sore but the muscle is still tight. This means that the trigger point is still lurking in the background and will likely resurface at some point. In this case, it's a good idea to continue work on turning these trigger points, as this will greatly improve your flexibility and muscle health.

When treating latent triggers, you can be more aggressive than when treating active ones. Latent triggers can also be made inactive through consistent stretching and by getting fitter and stronger. After the initial treatment, stretching and building strength helps make your triggers less responsive, making them less prone to flare-ups.

Neural Compression & Trigger Points

There are three types of pain: somatic pain (which comes from the joints in the body), visceral pain (which comes from the organs in the body), and neuropathic pain (which comes from nerves in the body).

Somatic pain arises from trigger points. It might even create somatic referred pain, where you feel pain across a broader area around the trigger point. However, trigger points can also compress nerves, leading to neuropathic pain.

You've probably experienced neuropathic pain before. It's that numbing and tingling sensation you feel when you hit your funny bone. It kind of feels like a shooting pain. When a muscle goes into spasm due to a trigger point, you experience somatic pain but if the spastic muscle presses on a nerve, you can also experience neuropathic pain.

However, this only happens in areas where muscles run across the same spaces that nerves run through, which means this only occurs when trigger points impact three specific muscles in the body including the scalenes, the pectoralis minor, and the piriformis.

The scalenes are located on each side of the neck. These muscles run across the nerves that come from the neck. Thus, when they are irritated and spasming, they can squeeze these nerve roots, creating neuropathic pain through the shoulders and arms. You can even feel weakness in the areas that the nerves innervate. The same thing happens when the pectoralis minor muscle spasms.

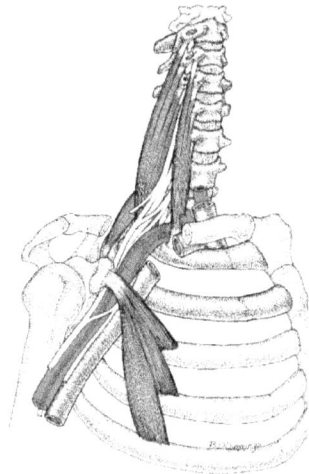

The nerve bundle to the arm running between the scalene muscles

The piriformis, on the other hand, impacts the sciatic nerve. When the piriformis has trigger points and spasms, you can experience shooting pain through the buttocks and down the legs. However, by addressing your trigger points in your piriformis muscle, you can eliminate both somatic and neuropathic pain.

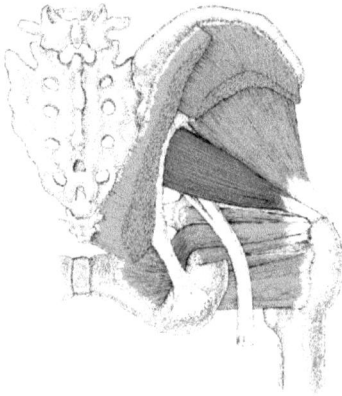

The sciatic nerve running past the piriformis muscle

It's important to take note of the above since neural pain can also be attributed to other conditions, such as a slipped disc. This means that trigger point therapy won't necessarily help eliminate your neuropathic pain. You may need other therapies or treatment to experience noticeable improvements. Usually, image testing can help determine the potential cause of your neuropathic pain.

Trigger Point Therapy: The Basics

In this section, we'll review how to find your trigger points and the steps involved in eliminating them. So, let's get straight to it. How can you perform trigger point therapy to relieve your pain?

Step 1: Finding Your Triggers

Trigger points can occur in any muscle in the body. However, the principles involved in finding your trigger points remain the same.

Initially, you want to figure out the direction of the muscle fibers. For example, the forearm muscles run from your elbow toward your hand. Thus, the muscle fibers also run in this direction.

Once you have figured out the direction of the muscle fibers, you can, then, run your fingers perpendicular to that direction, gently rubbing backwards and forwards, to find a tight band within the muscle.

Usually, this tight band is found in the biggest part of the muscle. As you move your fingers backwards and forwards, you will feel your skin move which indicates that the skin is free and separate from your fascia, which is a thin connective tissue that covers your muscles and nerve endings.

Along this band, you will find your trigger point. You'll know this since the area will be much more tender, sore, and firm than other parts on this tight band. As you press on this area, you will feel the trigger point activate and experience increased pain.

Step 2: Ischemic Pressure Treatment

Ischemic pressure helps to decrease blood flow and desensitizes the muscle spindles in this area, putting a stop to the pain loop your body is stuck in.

Once you've found your trigger point, press until it hurts. From there, you can determine how hard to press so that you're just below that pain threshold. Essentially, you want enough pressure to irritate the trigger point but not enough to hurt. Once you've found that pressure, hold for 20 to 30 seconds. This causes the trigger point to go to sleep.

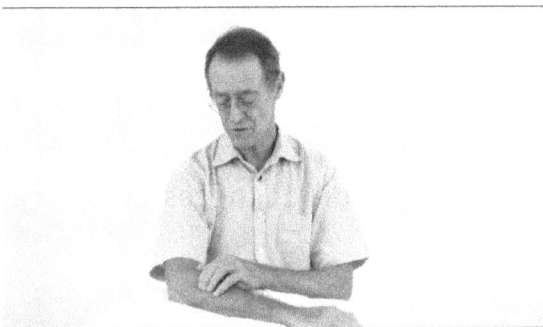

Ischemic pressure treatment #1

After the initial 20 to 30 seconds, you can, then, push slightly harder for another 20 to 30 seconds. You should notice the pain and tenderness becoming softer and softer, until it's basically melting away. This means you've effectively turned off the trigger point.

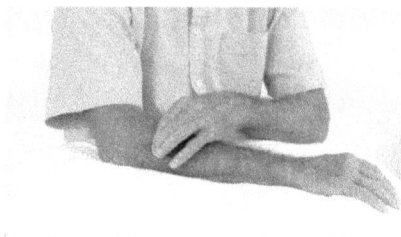

Ischemic pressure treatment #2

Most trigger points require a total of 90 seconds of ischemic pressure. Again, this process shouldn't necessarily cause increased pain. For every pressure level, you want to apply just enough pressure so that you are slightly above your pain threshold.

Step 3: Perform a Neuromuscular Stretch

While you've effectively turned off the trigger, the muscle is still shortened. Thus, the next step to permanently eliminate your pain involves stretching the muscle so that it returns to its original length.

Yet, if you stretch the area too quickly, you turn the muscle spindles back on and end up reactivating the trigger point. This is why you have to stretch the area in a specific way — known as neuromuscular stretching.

Neuromuscular stretching involves the use of your breath. Your breath is intricately linked to part of the nervous system called the autonomic nervous system. The autonomic nervous system consists of two parts: the sympathetic and parasympathetic nervous systems.

The sympathetic nervous system is associated with the stress response, also known as your "fight-or-flight system." The parasympathetic system, on the other hand, is your "rest and digest system," which helps relieve tension and helps you relax.

Basically, you want to set yourself up to stretch the affected muscle. As you stretch, take a deep breath in, which should increase tension in the body, then count to six.

Gently breathe out, counting to nine or 10. At this stage, you should feel your body relax. As your body relaxes, you can gently stretch the muscle even further as your muscle spindles relax, allowing you to reach new limits with that particular muscle.

For example, when stretching the trapezius muscle, you start by sitting on your hand. You then use your opposite hand to gently pull your neck to your opposite side. Breathe in and count to six, then breathe out, count to nine or 10, and see if you can gently pull your head a little further to your opposite side.

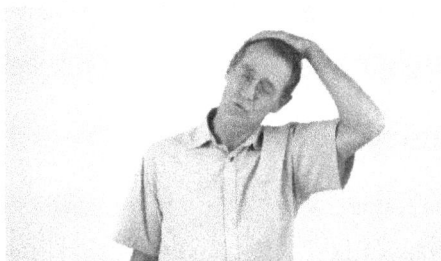

Neuromuscular stretch

Repeat this breathing process three times.

The key for this to work is to ensure you worked out which muscle your trigger point is located in. Throughout this book, there are pictures indicating points of pain and where common trigger points can be found. Use these pictures to help you determine which muscle your trigger point is located in.

If you experience difficulty with this, the best thing you can do is use your instincts. Go off of the information your body is giving you and what sensations you feel when you stretch or move a particular area of your body.

Step 4: Apply Heat

After you've completed your neuromuscular stretch, applying heat can further help relax the muscle and increase blood flow. For this step, you can use a heat pack, such as a wheat bag which you can buy or even make yourself.

Microwave your heat pack with a glass of water for two to five minutes. This helps to create a moist heat. Then, apply the heat pack to your affected area for 5 to 10 minutes. The area should have a bit of redness, signifying an increase in blood flow to the area.

Afterwards, perform a very gentle second stretch, which should help completely alleviate your pain and help you feel a world of difference.

Posture & Muscle Imbalances: Do They Play a Part?

With laptops and smartphones, many of us might find ourselves slouching and hunching forward throughout our workdays. Inevitably, this has led many more people to experience pain within their daily lives. In fact, poor posture can increase trigger point incidences, which is why becoming more aware of your posture is of the utmost importance.

Understanding Good Posture VS Bad Posture

Essentially, proper posture is the position where your body is experiencing the least amount of stress. Your spine consists of vertebrates that are stacked slightly differently and are designed to take up their specific position along your spinal curve. These positions make up correct posture, limiting the impact of gravity and minimizing the work your muscles have to do to keep you upright.

Along your spine, you have postural muscles, which have type 1 fibers consisting of lots of muscle spindles. These muscles help balance your joints so that you can hold yourself against gravity. In fact, your postural muscles are working almost all of the time. Yet, if your posture is bad, they have to do more work, which they aren't necessarily designed to do.

As you round your shoulders and protrude your neck forward, your posture collapses. The upper curves of the spine become more prominent, which means your neck and shoulder muscles have to do more work to keep you upright. This further increases pain, fatigue, and even headaches.

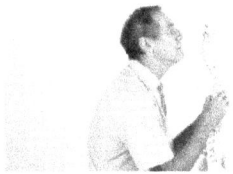

Poor posture - chin forward

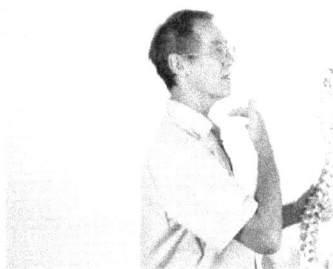

Good posture

These imbalances at the top of the spine also work their way down, adding more stress on the lower back. As a result, your lumbar, low back, curve might also increase to compensate for problems occurring at the top of the spine.

This changes your entire body and its function. Your body is, essentially, working against its innate design. This interferes with the flow of the body, creating various muscle imbalances and other issues

Fixing Your Posture

If you're prone to bad posture, setting reminders throughout your day can help you gain the awareness you need to prevent postural deficits.

Experts suggest that the point where the neck joins your head is the primary position you must train to improve overall posture and decrease imbalances throughout the body. When you improve the alignment of this area, everything else improves.

So, how can you do this? The best way is to imagine that there is a golden thread extending upward from the back of your head. This thread allows your head to float upwards and sit correctly on top of your neck.

When you assume this position, your chin also comes slightly down. In other words, your neck elongates and your chin slightly nods forward, which should cause any tension to disappear.

In this position, you can also perform a slight nodding movement with your head. The easiest way to do this is by using a mirror. To the side of the mirror, place your hand on the back of your head to maintain proper alignment, then gently nod the head, moving your chin down and up.

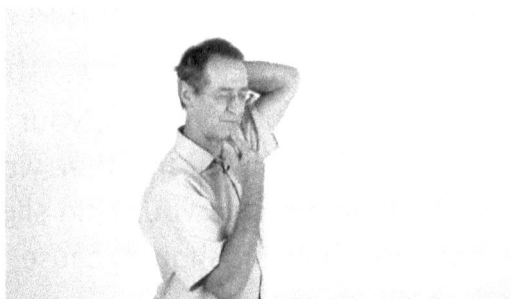

Posture Correction

This frees up that primary neck area, allowing everything below it to fall into proper alignment. Integrating this practice into your day-to-day is the best way to become more aware of your posture and to change the way your whole body stacks in relation to gravity.

How Often Should You Treat Trigger Points?

The truth is this depends.

For someone with trigger points everywhere, it's really important for them to recognize that their trigger points are part of a bigger pain problem. In these cases, the person has become overly sensitive to pain, which means the treatment approach slightly differs.

For example, if someone with many trigger points were to perform the trigger point therapy sequence above for all of their trigger points, they may actually end up amplifying their pain and create a worse situation. Instead, it's best to choose the two to four worst and most active areas for treatment.

This can help prevent whole-body flare-ups and help you determine if something worked or not, as well as what adjustments can be made. For instance, you might select your two worst trigger points, apply the treatment, then wait and see how you feel over the next couple of days. This allows you to figure out how much your body and pain system can take.

Meanwhile, for individuals experiencing trigger points in one localized area, they can likely be more aggressive with their treatment. At the same time, less is always best so that you avoid flare-ups. Always be gentle and sensitive to how you're feeling and how much you can get away with.

Some individuals with localized pain may be able to aggressively treat their area two to three times a day for consecutive days in a row and have their pain easily eliminated. Yet, again, listening to your body and taking a gentle approach is key.

Chapter 2: Head & Neck

Head & Neck Trigger Points

At some point in their life, around 50% of the world population will have significant neck pain. Yet, neck pain comes with a variety of different causes, frequently arising from the discs and the joints in the neck. At the same time, a very large proportion of neck pain comes from trigger points.

Tension headaches can further arise from tight occipitalis, frontalis, and suboccipital muscles. These three muscles, along with the trapezius muscle, are the main tension headache contributors.

Below, we explore techniques to effectively turn off the trigger points in the neck and eliminate your pain. We'll look at the trapezius in the shoulder section of this book.

Choosing the Correct Muscle to Treat

On the next page, you'll see pictures of the pain patterns created by trigger points in the head & neck muscles. This exercise is like picking suspects out of a lineup.

Find the one (or two) pain patterns that most match what you're feeling, and navigate to that muscle in this chapter.

Links to muscles:

Occipitalis Pterygoids Sternocleidomastoid

Frontalis   Scalenes   Masseter   Occipitais
Suboccipitals

The Occipitalis Muscle

The occipitalis muscle lies at the base of the skull, originating from the superior nuchal line of the occipital bone, which is a line that runs along the base of the skull, and inserting into the galea aponeurosis. If you feel for the occipitalis muscle, you'll find a little depression just beneath the muscle. In fact, this little muscle is what allows some people to wiggle their ears.

The occipitalis and frontalis muscle actually act together, counterbalancing one another. For example, when you raise eyebrows (an action of the frontalis muscle), the occipitalis muscle will also slightly contract as part of this movement.

With chronic anxiety, the occipitalis muscles frequently cause tension, as do the frontalis muscles. Thus, for individuals with anxiety, these are great muscles to target and relax.

Pterygoids   Temporalis

Sternocleidomastoid   Frontalis

Scalenes   Masseter

Suboccipitals   Occipitals

You'll see this muscle in the picture below. Usually, a trigger point in the occipitalis muscle is right in the middle of the muscle. With occipitalis trigger points, you may also experience in the top and front of your head.

Occipitals Trigger Point

Treating Occipitalis Trigger Points

When finding the occipitalis muscle, you'll want to locate the nuchal ridge. To do this, simply run your hand up to the base of the skull until you feel a ledge, then run your hand parallel toward the ear. About two centimeters up from this, you'll feel a little depression, which is where you'll find the occipital muscle.

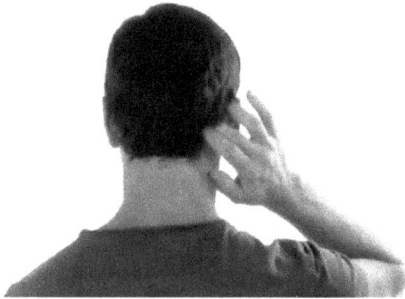

Occipitals Treatment

Usually, you'll find the trigger point right in the center of the depression. In order to find the trigger point, you can simply move your finger back and forth until you find that sore spot.

Once found, use your middle finger to support your index finger, then press into it, applying ischemic pressure. This involves applying enough pressure to irritate the trigger point but not enough to hurt.

Once you've found that pressure, hold for 20 to 30 seconds. After the initial 20 to 30 seconds, you can, then, push slightly harder for another 20 to 30 seconds.

You should notice the pain and tenderness becoming softer and softer, until it's basically melting away. This means you've effectively turned off the trigger point. Most trigger points require a total of 90 seconds of ischemic pressure.

Since this muscle is so small, it's difficult to do any other treatment, such as stretching or cold or heat therapy.

The Frontalis Muscle

The frontalis muscle is the small muscles in front of the forehead. Its origin is the galea aponeurotica and its insertion is the orbicularis oculi muscle. They work as part of your facial expressions, allowing you to raise your eyebrows. Similar to the occipitalis muscles, the frontalis muscles usually only have one trigger point.

Trigger points in the frontalis muscle typically cause localized pain and feel like a headache over the eye. They are usually located in the second wrinkle of the forehead above the eyebrow, as illustrated in the picture below. Tightness in this muscle can also lead to tension headaches. So, how can you treat it?

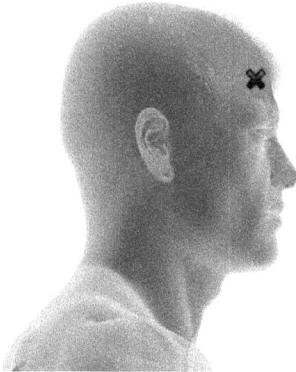

Frontalis Trigger Point

Treating Frontalis Trigger Points

Find the trigger point by using your index finger and moving it backwards and forwards. Focus on the area that is tender, then push hard enough so that you feel pain. You can place your middle finger on the top of your index finger for extra support here.

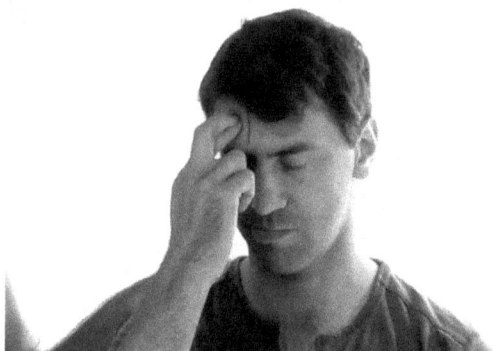

Frontalis Trigger Treatment

Then, you'll want to reduce pressure so that you are just below the pain threshold. From there, you can apply ischemic pressure, which starts with holding this pressure for 20 to 30 seconds. After the initial 20 to 30 seconds, you can push slightly harder for another 20 to 30 seconds.

You should notice the pain and tenderness becoming softer and softer, until it's basically melting away. This means you've effectively turned off the trigger point. Most trigger points require a total of 90 seconds of ischemic pressure.

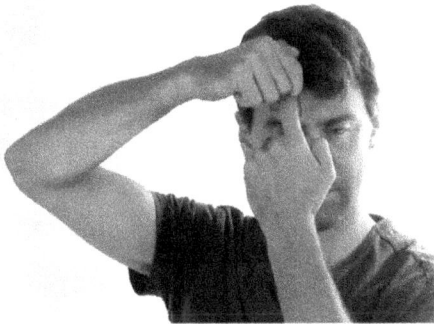

Since the frontalis muscle is so small and runs across a bone, you can't stretch it as you would bigger muscles. However, you can use myofascial release to stretch it. To do this, place both of your index fingers on the tender point, then press your fingers away from each other. You can support your fingers by leaning your knuckles on one another and using them as a lever. Hold this stretch for about 20 seconds.

Frontalis Stretch

After you've completed the stretch, you can then use hot and cold therapy to further alleviate tension and pain in this area. Take a cold pack and apply it to where the muscle starts near the eyebrows and gently glide the ice upwards along the skin.

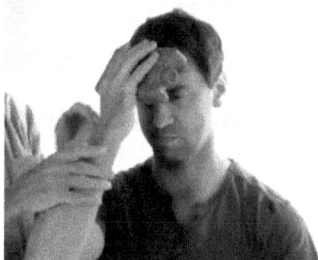

Frontalis cold treatment

This cold acts as a distraction, which further turns off the trigger point. Do this motion about 2 to 3 times.

You can then follow this cold therapy with heat, such as a wheat bag. Apply the heat to the area for at least 5 minutes. When you remove the heat, you should notice the area is red. This means there is increased blood flow, which can help encourage healing.

The Lateral & Medial Pterygoid Muscles

The lateral and medial pterygoid muscles are complex controllers of your jaw. These muscles cause the jaw joint to glide side to side and forward and back. Triggers in these muscles can contribute to jaw joint pain, often known as temporomandibular joint disorder or TMJ pain.

In these muscles, trigger points are often hidden and tough to get to. The lateral pterygoid muscle actually has two divisions, the inferior and superior divisions, as shown in the picture below.

These muscles work to contract and pull the condyle forward and toward the midline of the body, as well as across to the opposite side.

Usually, there are two significant triggers in this muscle, one in the inferior portion and one in the superior portion. In the medial pterygoid muscle, there is often one trigger point in the center of the muscle.

In fact, usually, the medial pterygoid muscle is secondary when it comes to causes of pain in the jaw joint. So, let's take a look at how to properly treat these triggers.

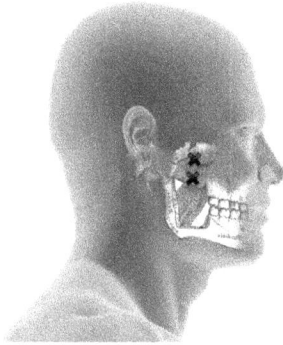

Lateral Pterygoid Trigger Points

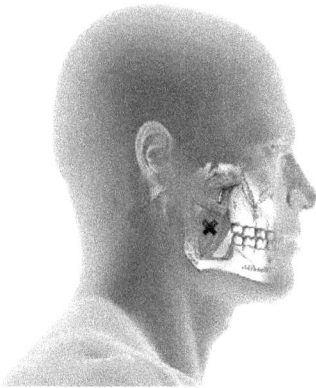

Medial Pterygoid Trigger Points

39

Treating Lateral & Medial Pterygoid Trigger Points

As previously mentioned, the trigger points in this muscle lie deep, which can make them difficult to get to. Basically, you want to feel for the head of the mandible and find the zygomatic arch, which is located in front of the ear. You can actually get better access to these muscles by placing something in your mouth and biting down on it, such as a thick cloth.

Once you find those trigger points in this area, you want to press into them and follow the ischemic pressure principles. This means applying just enough pressure so that you're below the pain threshold. Hold this pressure for 20 to 30 seconds.

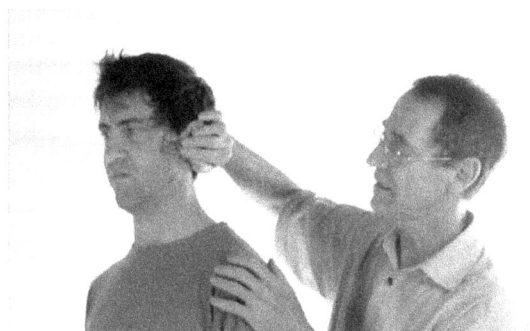

Pterygoid Treatment

After the initial 20 to 30 seconds, you can push slightly harder for another 20 to 30 seconds. You should notice the pain and tenderness becoming softer and softer, until it's basically melting away. This means you've effectively turned off the trigger point. Most trigger points require a total of 90 seconds of ischemic pressure.

Use cold therapy to turn off the triggers. The cold acts as a distraction. The key is to sweep it across the muscle. Start where the muscle originates, which is closer to the ear, and move forward toward the midline of the body, sweeping across your face. You should move at a pace of about 2 centimeters a second and perform at least 2 to 3 sweeps in total.

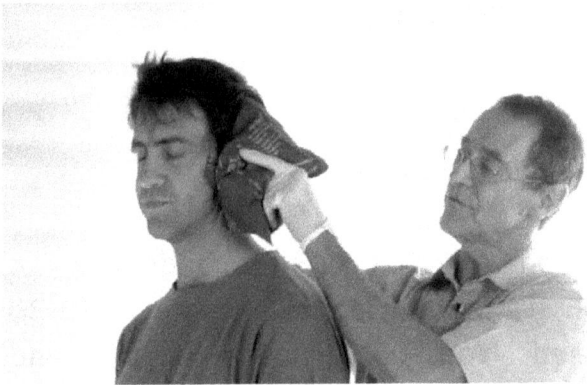

Pterygoid Cold Treatment

Unfortunately, myofascial release doesn't work for these muscles as they are limited by restraining ligaments. Thus, stretching comes down to performing the opposite movement of what the muscles do.

For the lateral pterygoid muscle, this means retracting the muscle and gently moving the jaw to one side, holding for about 20 to 30 seconds. Follow this sequence up with heat, leaving it for 5 minutes.

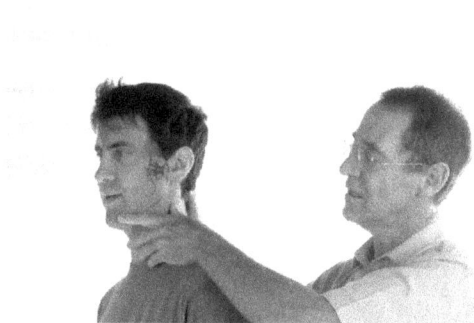

Pterygoids Stretch

For the medial pterygoid muscle, retract your jaw and hold for 20 to 30 seconds. This will stretch the muscle as best as you can. Afterwards, similar to the lateral pterygoid, apply heat for 5 to 10 minutes.

After the heat portion, you can relax and do the stretch again.

The Masseter

The masseter is a powerful muscle that is primarily used for closing the mouth and chewing. When you clench your teeth, you can actually feel this muscle slightly jump out from the jaw joint. This muscle originates from the zygomatic arch and inserts along the edge of the mandible. It has both superficial and deep components.

Trigger points are typically found in the center of this muscle. These points can refer pain to the jaw and cheek, as well as into the teeth and ear. You can find a total of six trigger points in this muscle, as illustrated in the picture below. These trigger points can become activated due to bruxism (a problem where one grinds their teeth), as well as from simple activities, such as sitting in the dentist chair for a long time with your mouth wide open.

These trigger points may lead to you not being able to open your mouth wide enough. Usually, the opening of the mouth measures about three knuckles. Yet, anything below this indicates a limited range of motion.

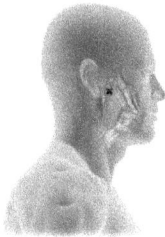

Masseter Trigger Points #1

Masseter Trigger Points #1

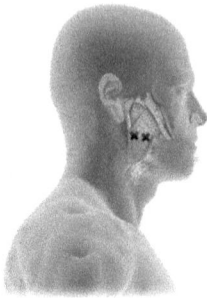

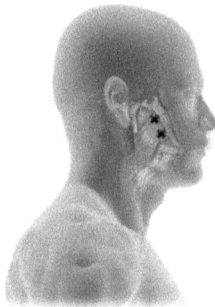

Masseter Trigger Points #3

Masseter Trigger Points #4

Treating Masseter Trigger Points

Use your index finger to run backwards and forwards along the muscle until you find the tender area. Once found, place the middle finger over your index finger for support, and gently reduce the pressure so that you're just below the pain threshold. Then, use the ischemic pressure principles outlined earlier in this book to deactivate the trigger point.

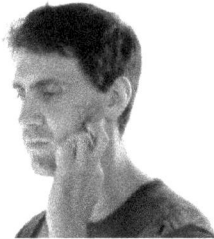

Masseter Ischemic Treatment

Alternatively, you can also place your finger into your mouth with your thumb on the outside and gently squeeze along the muscle until you find the trigger point. Once you find the trigger point, pin that part of the muscle, pressing in and using ischemic pressure.

Afterwards, use cold therapy by placing a cold pack at the jaw and moving it upwards along the muscle at about two centimeters per second. Do 2 to 3 sweeps, then stretch.

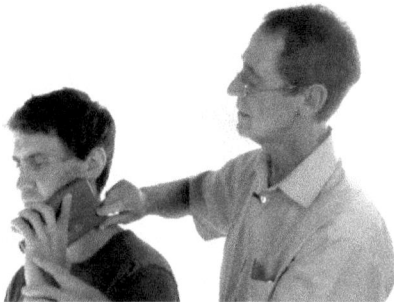

Masseter Cold Treatment

A stretch for the masseter is performed by hooking your index and middle finger on the lower teeth and opening your mouth. Bring your gaze up and head back, allowing your head to act as a counterbalance.

In this position, take a deep breath in, hold for a count of 6, then breath out and wait 2 to 3 seconds, allowing the masseter to relax. You should be able to lean into this stretch a bit more and repeat this breathing process for 2 to 3 rounds. For more of a stretch, you can also push the jaw gently forward.

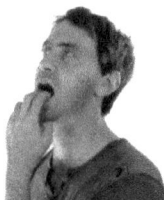

Masseter Stretch

Afterwards, place a heat pack on for 5 minutes or until the area is red. From there, you can do another stretch.

The Scalenes

The scalene muscles stabilize the neck against sidewards movement and help lift the first rib during forced breathing. These muscles are located between the sternocleidomastoid and upper trapezius, sitting in the sagittal plane of the body. This means if you were to cut the body in half, these muscles sit almost right where you would make that cut.

Scalene muscle triggers are frequently caused by pulling, lifting, or tugging. They can also arise due to chronic coughing. Triggers in this area can cause pain in the chest, upper thoracic spine, arm, and hand. They can further lead to nerve entrapment of the brachial plexus branch, leading to pain, numbness, and weakness in the arm and hand.

The anterior and medial scalenes is the most common spot to get trigger points, as illustrated in the picture below. Infrequent trigger points can also be found in the posterior scalenes. You'll know your trigger points are located in this muscle if you go to lift your arm over your head and the pain disappears. So, let's look into how you can treat this area.

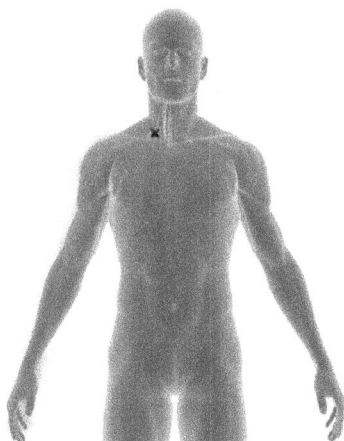

Scalene Trigger Point #1

Scalenes Trigger Point #2

Treating Scalene Trigger Points

For finding trigger points in the scalene muscles, lay on your side with the affected side facing upwards. This is important so that if you accidentally press too hard on your carotid artery and feel faint or dizzy, you won't fall over and hurt yourself.

Gently press with your index fingers into the muscle until you find the sensitive and tender spot. Once found, use the ischemic pressure principles to deactivate the trigger point. Afterwards, you can use heat. In fact, you should use heat after ischemic pressure, cold therapy, and stretching for 5 minutes at a time.

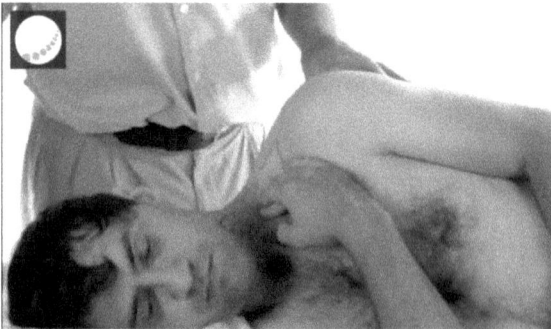

Scalene Ischemic Pressure Treatment

From there, you can use cold starting at the neck and running down the arm, sweeping at about 2 centimeters per second. Do three to four sweeps. Again, this can help distract the trigger point, allowing for further deactivation.

Afterwards, you can perform a stretch of the scalenes. This involves slightly tilting the head back and to one side. Your gaze should be directed upwards. Hold your

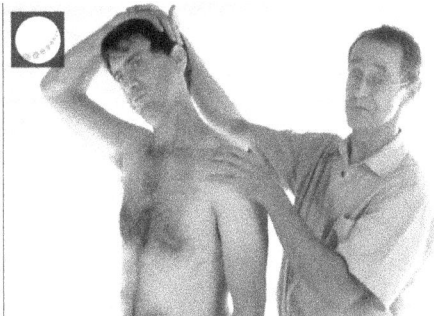

hand on your head and use the neuromuscular technique for breathing to allow for a greater release. Again, afterwards, you can apply heat for 5 minutes.

Scalenes Stretch

The Sternocleidomastoid

The Sternocleidomastoid is an important muscle in your neck, helping flex and rotate your head. It's also one of the more complicated muscles to treat because it has two branches or divisions to it – the sternal division and the clavicular division. These two divisions move the head in quite different directions, but are still branches of the same muscle.

Trigger points in the sternocleidomastoid can arise due to stress breathing, bad posture, and working with your head turned for a long time. This can result in referred pain toward the back of the head, pain in the ear, pain across the face or cheek, dizziness, abnormalities with depth perception, tinnitus, jaw pain, and symptoms similar to trigeminal neuralgia.

In the sternocleidomastoid, there are four triggers in the most superficial division and three triggers in the deeper division, as illustrated in the picture below. So, let's examine how to treat this muscle and eliminate your pain.

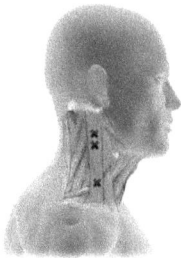

Sternocleidomastoid Triggers #1

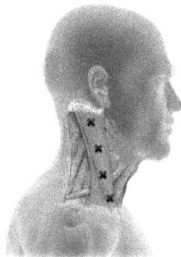

Treating Sternocleidomastoid Trigger Points

Feel up and down the neck, squeezing the muscle between two fingers, until you find your trigger point. This will be a really tender and painful spot on the muscle. Stop here and press hard enough so that you're just below the pain threshold. Use ischemic principles to deactivate the trigger point, followed by heat for 5 minutes.

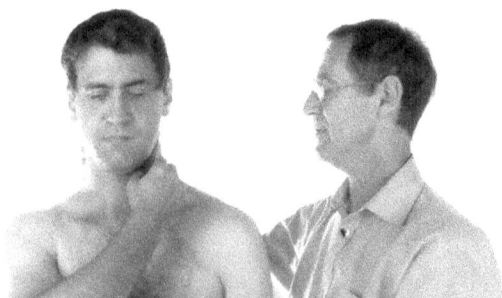

Sternocleidomastoid Ischemic Treatment #1

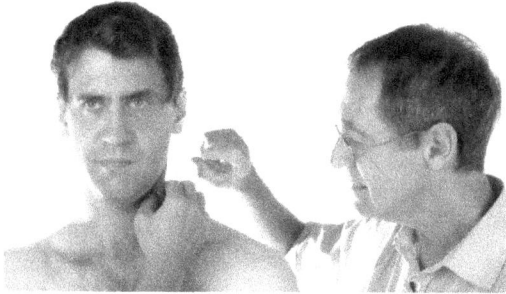

Sternocleidomastoid Ischemic Treatment #2

You can then use cold therapy as a distraction to further turn off this trigger point. Start with the ice pack at the lowest part of the muscle and move up toward where the pain is located, such as on the forehead, and perform 2 to 3 sweeps. Again, use heat for 5 minutes here.

From there, you can stretch the sternal and clavicular divisions of the sternocleidomastoid muscle.

For the sternal division, turn your head toward the affected side, keeping your head vertical and your shoulders relaxed. Hold your head by using your hand to maintain your chin position. Then, use the neuromuscular techniques to maximize

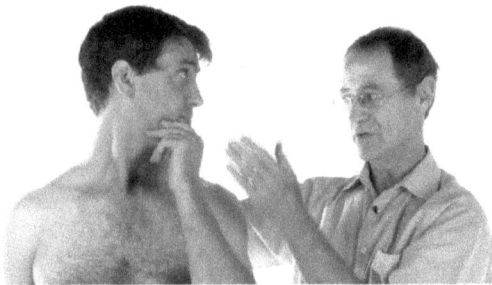

this stretch.

Sternocleidomastoid Stretch Sternal Division

For the clavicular division, bring your head to the opposite side of the trigger points, bringing your gaze slightly up. Use your hand to hold your head here, and utilize neuromuscular techniques and breathing to further relax and stretch the clavicular division.

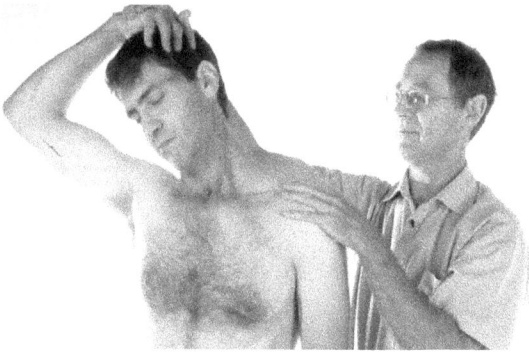

Sternocleidomastoid Stretch Clavicular Division

After stretching, you can, again, apply heat for 5 minutes.

The Suboccipitals

The suboccipitals are located below the occipital bones at the base and back of the head, originating lower and inserting at the superior and inferior nuchal line. These are very important small posture muscles that balance the head and allow your brain to know the position of your head in space.

They also help with rotating and extending the head. Triggers in these muscles are a quite common cause of tension headaches – they cause a pain deep in your head.

Four trigger points can be found in each of the four divisions of this muscle on each side of the head. In fact, you might not necessarily feel these triggers unless you're applying pressure, since pain is often quite broad, such as in the case of a tension headache. Typically, these trigger points are caused by whiplash or bad posture. So, how can you address these?

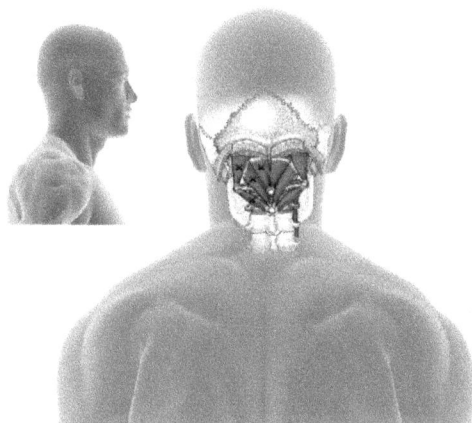

Suboccipitals Trigger Points

Treating Suboccipital Trigger Points

Use your ring or index finger to feel along the edge of the nuchal line. Once you find a painful and tender spot, use ischemic pressure principles to deactivate the trigger point.

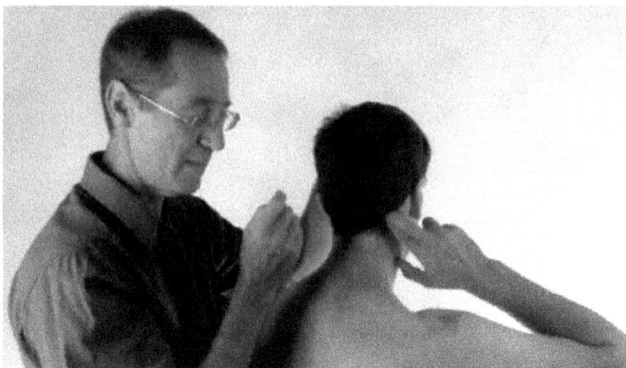

Suboccipitals Ischemic Treatment

Now that you've switched off the trigger point, you want to stretch. To do this, take one hand and place it over the back of your head with your fingers pointing down.

Suboccipitals Stretch

Take your other hand and place it on your chin, with your fingers pointing up. Gently push your chin towards your chest, until you feel a slight stretch in the lower part of the back of your head. Use the neuromuscular stretching principles to achieve an even deeper stretch.

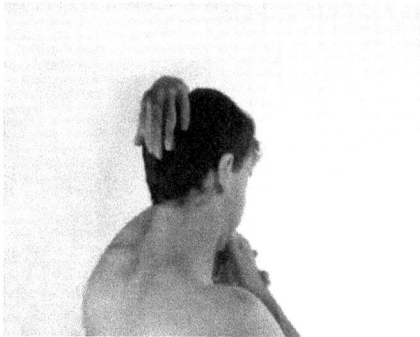

The Temporalis Muscle

The temporalis is a muscle that helps with chewing – it pulls your mouth closed. It's a fan-shaped muscle next to your ear. It refers pain down to your teeth, which can be a confusing problem for dentists and patients alike.

The temporalis muscle has a broad attachment along the side of the skull, with the tendon tucking under the zygomatic arch. When it contracts, it pulls upwards and closes the jaw.

Within this muscle, you can find up to 4 trigger points. So, let's look closer at how you can find these triggers and eliminate them.

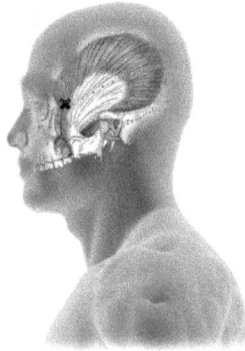

Temporalis Trigger Points #1

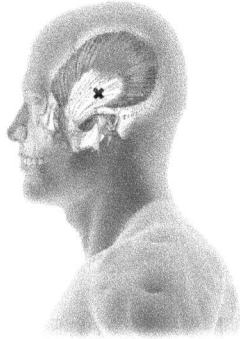

Temporalis Trigger Points #2

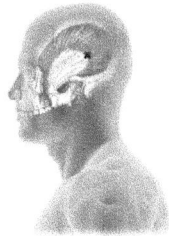

Temporalis Trigger Points #3

Treating Temporalis Trigger Points

Gently clench your teeth so that you can find the muscle bulging beneath your hair. Feel for a tight band and find that tender trigger point. Apply ischemic pressure principles until the trigger is turned off.

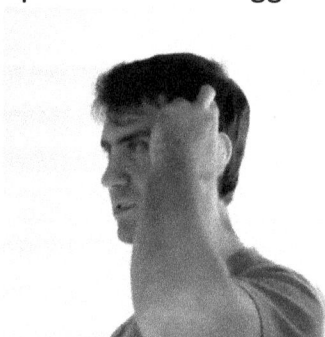

Temporalis Treatment

You can then use a cold pack to further distract the trigger point. Start at the origin of the muscle and move downwards along the jaw at a pace of about 2 centimeters per second. Perform 2 to 3 sweeps.

Then, you'll also want to stretch the temporalis muscle. Do this by gently opening your mouth and hooking your fingers over your bottom teeth. Bring your head slightly backwards and open your jaw as far as you can.

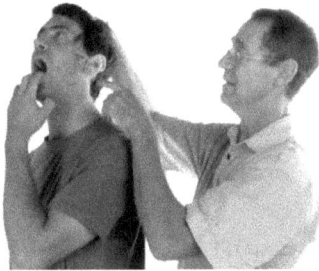

Temporalis Stretch

Use neuromuscular stretching and breathing to achieve a greater release, then apply heat for 5 minutes.

Chapter 3: Shoulder

Shoulder & Upper Back Trigger Points

E very year, 25% of individuals experience shoulder pain. This isn't surprising since the shoulder is actually a very mobile and complex joint used frequently in a person's day-to-day life.

There are various muscles involved in the movement of the shoulder. Below, we explore the techniques for each of these muscles, helping you turn off your trigger points in the shoulder and upper back and live a pain-free life.

Choosing the Correct Muscle to Treat

On the next page, you'll see pictures of the pain patterns created by trigger points in the shoulder muscles. This exercise is like picking suspects out of a lineup.

Find the one (or two) pain patterns that most match what you're feeling, and navigate to that muscle in this chapter.

Links to muscles:

Deltoids | Infraspinatus | Levator Scapulae | Latissimus Dorsi | Iliocostalis | Rhomboids | Subscapularis | Supraspinatus | Teres Minor | Upper Trapezius

The Deltoids

The deltoids are the power muscles of the shoulder. They are a triangle-shaped muscle, originating from the clavicle and scapula and attaching to the humerus.

This muscle covers the entire front of your shoulder joint, and consists of 5 main trigger points.

Three of these trigger points are found on the anterior and central portion. Meanwhile two of these trigger points are found on the posterior deltoid, as illustrated in the picture below. Pain is usually local, slightly radiating down the arm.

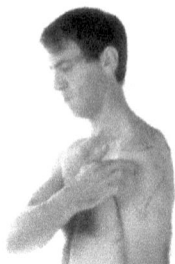

Anterior Deltoid Trigger Points

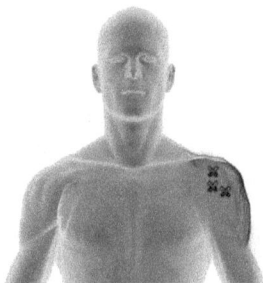

Posterior Deltoid Trigger Points

Treating Deltoid Trigger Points

Use your index finger to search for the sore area. Make sure while you do this that you relax your arm, allowing gravity to pull down on your limb. Once you locate your trigger point, use the ischemic pressure principles to eliminate your trigger point.

Deltoid Ischemic Treatment

For this muscle, you can also use a theracane to help target those hard-to-reach areas. Hold the theracane in your opposite hand and follow the same steps outlined above using the end of the theracane.

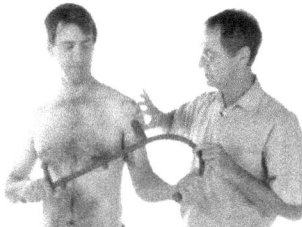

Deltoid Theracane Treatment

The second part of treating the deltoid trigger points involves stretching the muscle. The posterior and anterior portions of the deltoid require two different stretches.

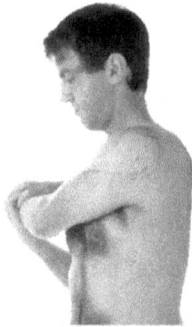

Posterior Deltoid Stretch

For the posterior deltoid, bring your arm forward and across your body, using your opposite hand to gently pull. You should feel a stretch on the back of your shoulder. You can then use neuromuscular breathing techniques to fully stretch and relax the muscle.

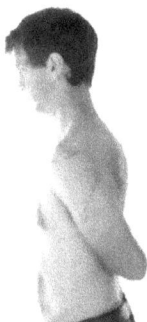

Anterior Deltoid Stretch

For the side and front of the deltoid, bring your arm behind your back with the elbow bent. Gently use your other hand to pull and lift up, allowing for a nice stretch on the front of the shoulder. Again, use neuromuscular breathing techniques to fully relax and stretch the muscle.

Afterwards, you can apply heat for 5 minutes.

The Infraspinatus Muscle

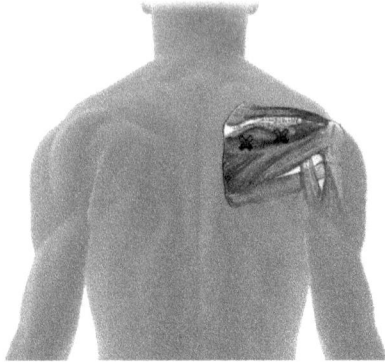

The infraspinatus muscle is a small muscle that belongs to the rotator cuff muscle group. It attaches on the inner edge of the shoulder blade and also to the humerus, as shown in the picture below.

The infraspinatus muscle triggers refer pain down the arm, into the neck and into the upper back. It's an important posture muscle and is very prone to triggers. You can find 3 trigger points within this muscle.

Usually, the trigger point closer to the spine will produce a deep ache along the thoracic spine. The other trigger points will often produce a deep ache down the shoulder and on the lower part of the neck.

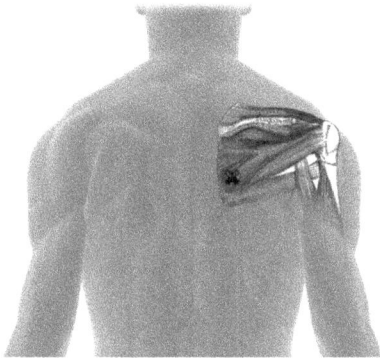

Infraspinatus Triggers #1

Infraspinatus Trigger Points #2

Treating Infraspinatus Trigger Points

Use your fingers to find the trigger points, pressing until you feel pain. Alternatively, you can also use a theracane or a tennis ball lying face up on it to apply ischemic pressure principles.

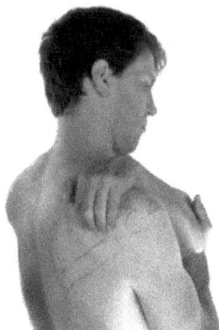

Infraspinatus Ischemic Treatment

Infraspinatus Theracane

Then, you can use cold therapy to further distract and eliminate your trigger point. Start next to the medial border of the scapula (close to the spine) and run the cold pack over the muscle and triggers and down the pain zone (usually the arm). You can, then, perform about 2 to 3 sweeps.

To finish off your treatment, you'll want to stretch this muscle. The easiest way to do this is by using a towel (if needed). Hold the towel in your opposite hand and bring your hand up behind your head, allowing the towel to hang.

Bring your affected side's hand behind your back and grab the bottom of the towel. Gently pull up and use neuromuscular stretching techniques to achieve a full release. Afterwards, you can apply heat and repeat this stretch, if needed.

The Latissimus Dorsi Muscle

The latissimus dorsi muscle is found in the lower two-thirds of the trunk of the body. It pulls the arm backwards and rotates it inwards. It's what you use when you go swimming, chop wood, perform chin ups, and do other powerlifting moves.

There are 2 trigger points in this muscle, as illustrated below, which refer pain into the shoulder and arm and also cause local pain in the back. These also usually cause a deep pain along the side of the spine and mid back. So, let's find out how you can eliminate these triggers!

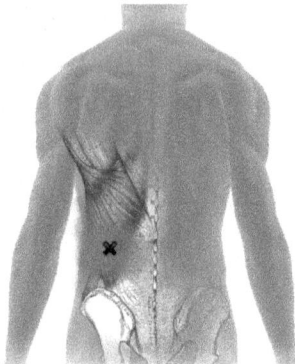

Latissimus Dorsi Trigger Points #1

Latissimus Dorsi Trigger Points #2

Treating Latissimus Dorsi Trigger Points

There are a few ways you can identify the triggers in this muscle. The first is by reaching your opposite hand back and digging into the muscle with your fingers to find that tender and painful spot.

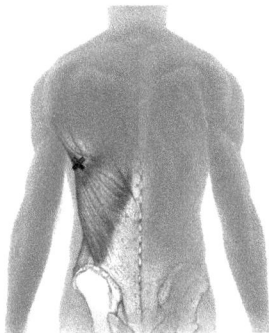

Latissimus Dorsi Ischemic Treatment

Alternatively, you can use the theracane, resting your affected side arm's on the cane and using your opposite arm to maneuver the cane, or you can use a tennis ball and lie on it face-up while rolling your body slightly onto your side to find your trigger point. Once you find your trigger point, use the ischemic principles to turn it off.

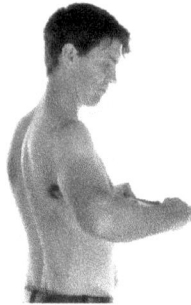

Latissimus Dorsi Theracane Treatment

From here, you can use cold therapy. However, you will need someone else to perform this part of the treatment (if possible). Your friend or partner should start with the ice pack at the origin of the muscle at the bottom of the back. They can then gently sweep the cold pack upwards and into the pain zone at about a

2 to 3 centimeter per second pace. Have them perform 2 to 3 sweeps.

After this, perform a stretch by bringing your arm up, bending your elbow, and allowing your hand to fall behind your head.

Latissimus Dorsi Stretch

Use your opposite hand to help with this stretch as you use neuromuscular stretching and breathing to fully stretch and relax the muscle.

The Levator Scapulae Muscle

The levator scapulae is a posture muscle. It's located along the side of the neck, inserting into the first 4 vertebrae and into the scapula (shoulder blade), as illustrated in the picture below. It lifts your shoulder and slightly turns your neck.

Triggers in this muscle cause pain locally in the shoulder and up into the neck. Yet, the central area of pain is between the scapula and lower neck. Often, someone will report feelings of stiffness and difficulty rotating their head to the side.

Essentially, there are two main trigger points in this muscle. One is located where the muscle attaches to the superior border of the scapula, and the second is located halfway up the muscle (usually underneath the trapezius so you need to dig to find it).

Levator Scapulae Trigger Points

Treating Levator Scapulae Trigger Points

Use your opposite hand to check for

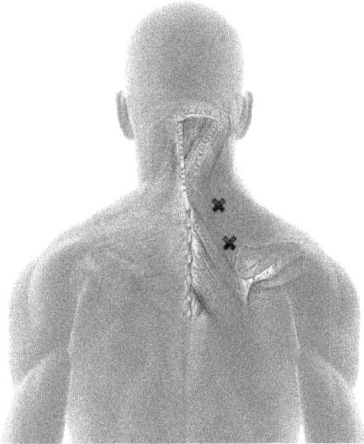

triggers along your levator scapulae. Search for that tender area, then apply ischemic pressure to turn off the trigger point. For easier access to these trigger points, you may need to slightly bend your neck, bringing your head slightly your shoulder.

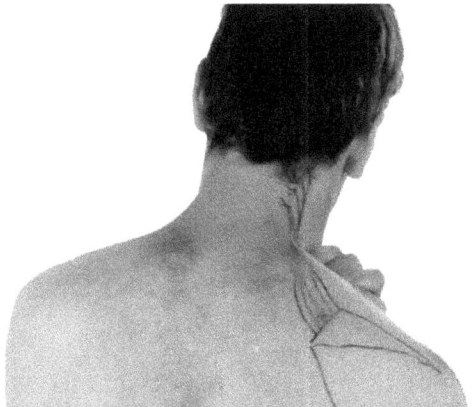

Levator Scapulae Ischemic Pressure

Follow ischemic pressure principles with cold therapy. Apply the cold below the muscle and move upwards over the muscle, moving it at a pace of about 2 centimeters per second. Perform 2 to 3 sweeps. You may find it easier to have someone do this for you as to avoid tension in the body.

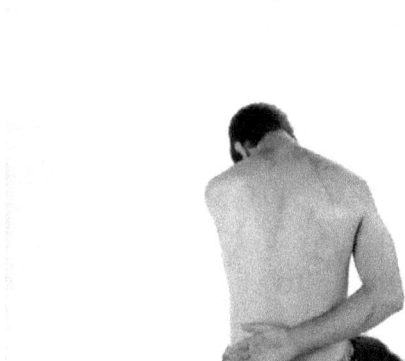

Levator Scapulae Stretch

From there, you can stretch the muscle to elongate the muscle which has likely become shortened by the trigger points. Gently bring your gaze toward your opposite armpit, placing your hand on your head to slightly pull when and if needed. Place your other hand behind your back. Then, use neuromuscular techniques and breathing to fully elongate the muscle.

Afterwards, apply heat for 5 minutes. It's probably best to lie down when you do this to allow your body to fully relax.

The Longissimus & Iliocostalis Muscles

These muscles run parallel to your spine. They run all the way from the pelvis to your neck and are posture muscles that keep you upright. The iliocostalis also helps you twist your spine. The longissimus muscle runs closer to the spine and the iliocostalis muscle runs right beside it, as illustrated in the picture.

The iliocostalis muscle has 3 triggers, whereas the longissimus has 2 main triggers (shown in the picture). The triggers located in the mid-back cause pain locally. The upper and lower triggers refer down the iliocostalis muscle into your buttock or up into your neck. So, let's find out how you can rid yourself of this pain and say goodbye to those triggers for good.

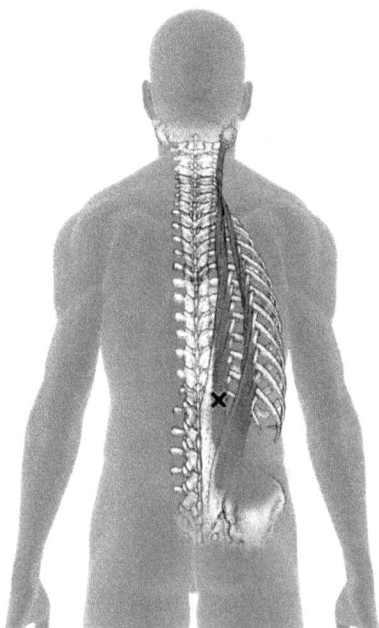

Longissimus Trigger Points #1

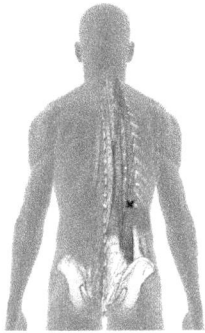

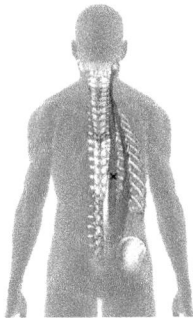

Longissimus Trigger Points #2

Iliocostalis Trigger Points #1

Iliocostalis Trigger Points #2

Iliocostalis Trigger Points #3

Treating Longissimus & Iliocostalis Trigger Points

For treating these areas, you will need a theracane. This is the primary use of this tool. It helps you reach areas that you simply can't reach with your hands.

Use your opposite hand to push the theracane in and rest your affected side's arm on the theracane. Tilt and move the tool until you find that tender spot. Once there, apply ischemic principles to turn off the trigger point.

Longissimus Theracane Treatment #1

Longissimus Theracane Treatment #2

For cold therapy, start where the muscle inserts and go over the pain zone. For example, if your pain is toward the pelvis and buttocks, start above the trigger and sweep over and down across the pain zone. Perform 2 to 3 sweeps.

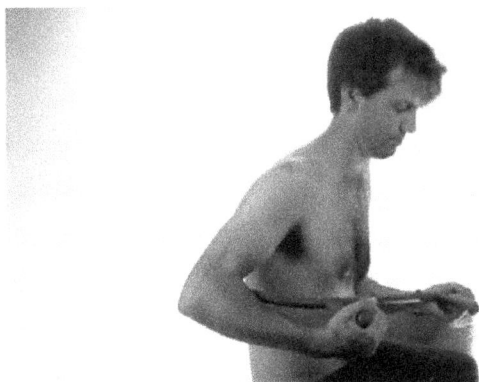

Afterwards, stretch the two muscles. For the longissimus, sit up with your legs straight in front of you and curl your spine

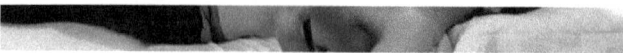

forward into a ball. Use neuromuscular principles and breathing to further lean into this stretch.

For the iliocostalis muscle, do the same thing but add a slight rotation, turning to the opposite side of where you felt pain and using neuromuscular principles to elongate the muscle as much as you can.

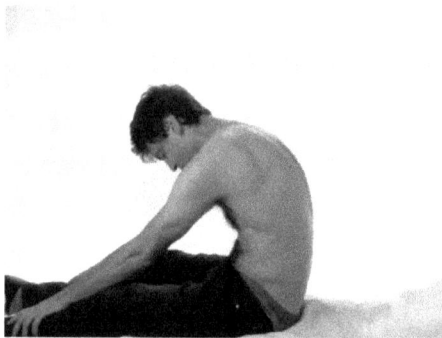

Longissimus Stretch

Finish off by applying heat for 5 minutes and performing another round of these stretches.

The Rhomboids

The rhomboid muscles are postural muscles that attach to the inner border of the scapula and run across the back, attaching to the spine. You use them when you pull back or hunch your shoulders. The three trigger points in this muscle, as illustrated in the picture, refer pain locally into the back of your shoulders, and these are really common sources of pain.

So, let's look at how you can go about treating rhomboid trigger points.

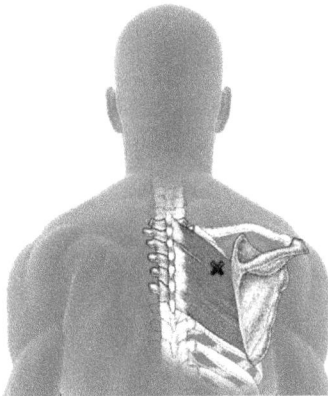

Rhomboid Trigger Points #1

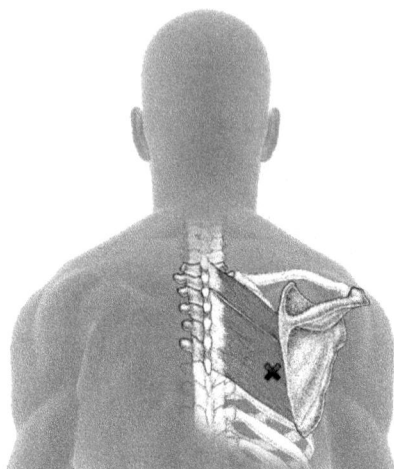

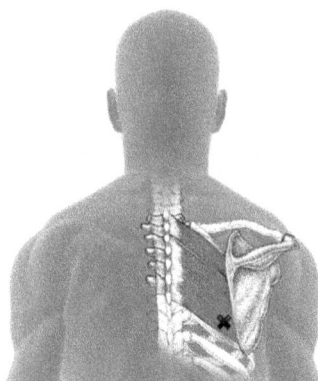

Rhomboid Trigger Points #2

Treating the Rhomboid Trigger Points

When it comes to identifying trigger points in the rhomboids, it can be difficult to determine if it is, in fact, the rhomboids or if it's the trapezius since both muscles run along the same area. However, it doesn't really matter since the technique is fairly the same. You can also choose to stretch both areas if you aren't sure.

Use the theracane to find your trigger points and press on it using ischemic pressure principles to turn it off. Alternatively,you can also use a tennis ball and move yourself up and down over top of it, modulating the amount of pressure you use.

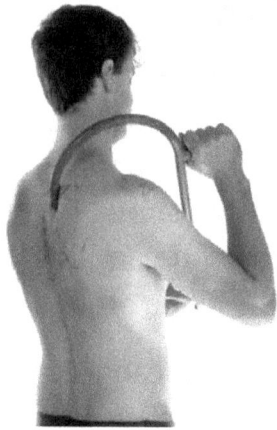

Rhomboids Theracane

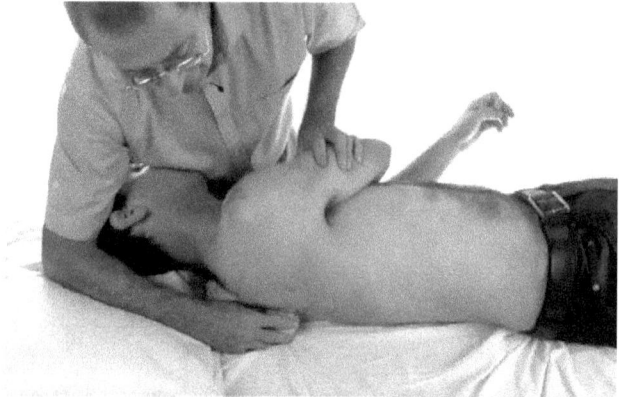

94

Rhomboids Tennis Ball Treatment

After completing the ischemic pressure principles, you can use cold to further distract the trigger point. For the rhomboids, start at the center and run the cold pack laterally over the muscle, covering the pain zone. Do this 2 to 3 times.

To stretch the muscle, protract your

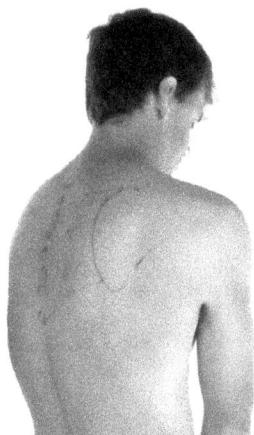

shoulder blades, curving your thoracic spine. Once you've reached the limit of this stretch, breathe in, hold for a count of

6, breath out, then wait 2 to 4 seconds for neuromuscular release.

Rhomboid Stretch

Repeat this process 2 to 3 times, then apply heat and stretch again.

The Subscapularis Muscle

The subscapularis is a hidden muscle. It's part of the rotator cuff muscle group, and it primarily protects and balances the head of the humerus as you move the shoulder joint.

This particular muscle is tucked between the shoulder blades and ribs, making it really hard to get to.

It has 3 trigger points, as shown in the picture, and these trigger points create pain primarily over the back of the shoulder joint, extending slightly over the scapula.

So, let's dive into how exactly you can access this muscle and eliminate trigger points.

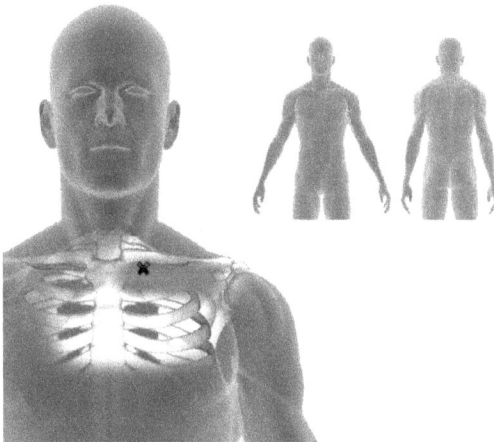

Subscapularis Trigger Points 1#

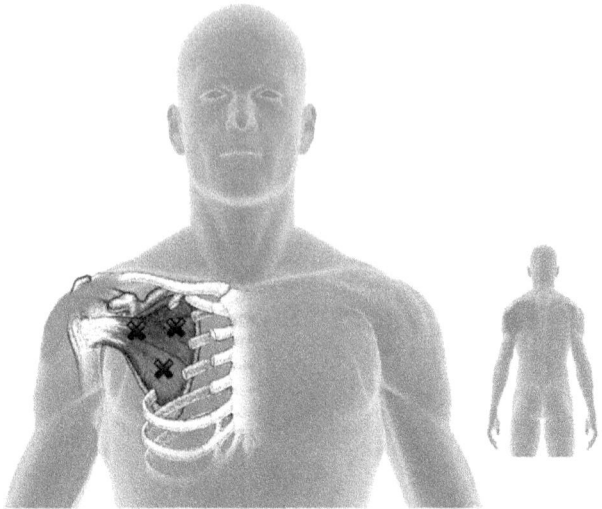

Subscapularis Trigger Points 2#

Treating Subscapularis Trigger Points

For access to this muscle, it's best if you lie on your side and lift your arm up over your head.

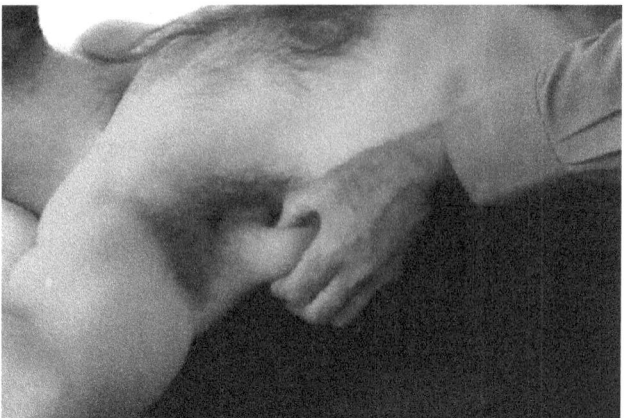

Subscapularis Muscle Location

This allows you to access in front of the scapula. Use your opposite hand (or a theracane) to feel for the edge of the scapula and locate the trigger points. Once found, use ischemic pressure principles to turn it off.

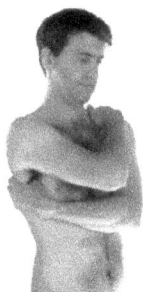

Subscapularis Ischemic Treatment

Subscapularis Theracane Treatment

You can then use cold, or have someone help you apply a cold pack. With your arm raised, apply the cold pack below the armpit, sweeping it upward and forward across the armpit and across the front of the shoulder joint. Do this 2 to 3 times.

Afterwards, you can stretch this muscle by fully flexing your arm over your head and bending your elbow, which internally rotates the shoulder, allowing your hand to fall backward behind your head.

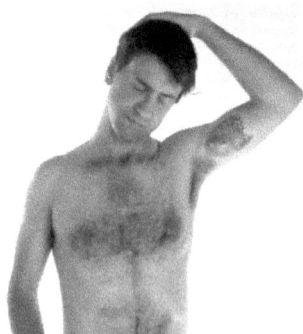

Subscapularis Stretch

This elongates the muscle, releasing any tightness and preventing that trigger point from becoming reactivated. Then, apply heat for 5 to 10 minutes and stretch again.

The Supraspinatus Muscle

This is a small posture muscle with a vital role. It moves, stabilizes, and balances the shoulder joint – along with the other rotator cuff muscles. This is a very mobile joint, and it is very prone to triggers.

As pictured, the supraspinatus attaches to the upper part of the shoulder blade and runs across the spine of the scapula to the head of the humerus. In rotator cuff injuries, the supraspinatus muscle is actually the primary tendon damaged. It further has 2 main trigger points, as illustrated. So, how can you eliminate your pain and trigger points in relation to this muscle?

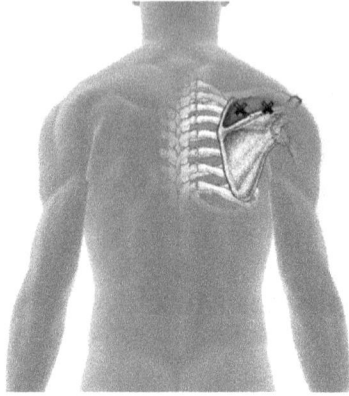

Supraspinatus Trigger Points

Treating Supraspinatus Trigger Points

Most individuals can reach this area with their opposite hand. You simply hook your fingers behind your shoulder and feel for that trigger point. If you struggle to reach it, you can use a theracane to find your trigger point and to apply ischemic pressure principles.

Supraspinatus Ischemic Treatment

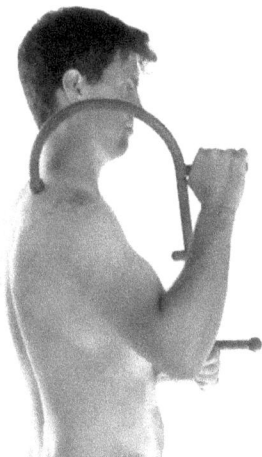

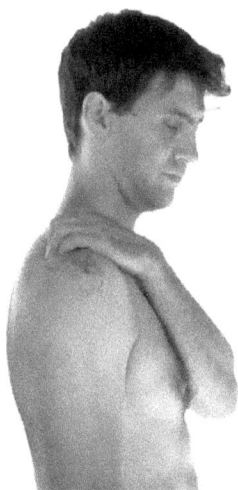

Supraspinatus Theracane

After you've used ischemic pressure to turn off the trigger point, you can further this by applying cold therapy. You may need a friend or partner to help you to do this properly. Start with the cold pack close to the spine and sweep across, at a 2 to 3 centimeters per second pace, toward the shoulder and down the arm. Do this 2 to 3 times.

Afterwards, perform a stretch by standing tall. Place your hand behind your back with your elbow bent. Use your other hand to gently pull your arm across and up your back, increasing extension and

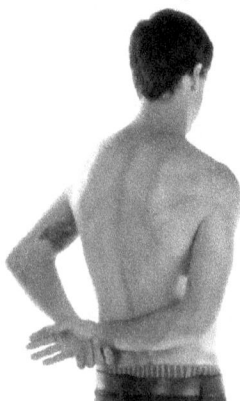

internal rotation of the arm.

Supraspinatus Stretch

Use the neuromuscular technique and breathing to increase this stretch and elongate the muscle. Then, apply heat for 5 to 10 minutes.

The Teres Minor Muscle

The teres minor arises from the back of the scapula and attaches just underneath the infraspinatus, which overlies part of this muscle. It then runs laterally outside of the scapula and attaches to the back and side of the humerus.

The function of this muscle is the same as the infraspinatus. They actually work in tandem. It's also a rotator cuff muscle that functions to balance the head of the humerus.

The teres minor has one trigger point along the lateral border of the scapula where it runs off of the glenohumeral joint. Pain from this trigger point is mainly felt over the lateral upper arm, radiating slightly down into the upper arm.

It usually feels like a deep and achy pain. So, let's look at how you can rid yourself of

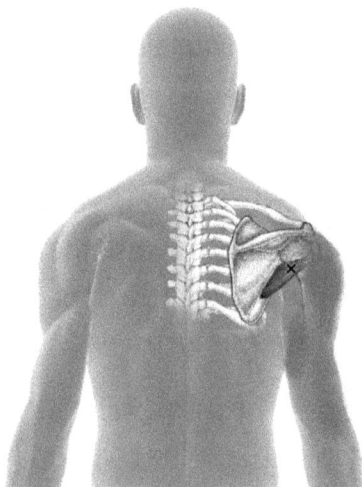

this pain!

Teres Minor Trigger Points

Treating Teres Minor Trigger Points

Using your opposite hand push hard slightly behind the shoulder joint. Once you've found that painful point, let the pressure off slightly so that you are just below the pain threshold. Then, use ischemic principles to turn off the trigger point. Alternatively, you can also use a theracane or tennis ball to find your trigger points.

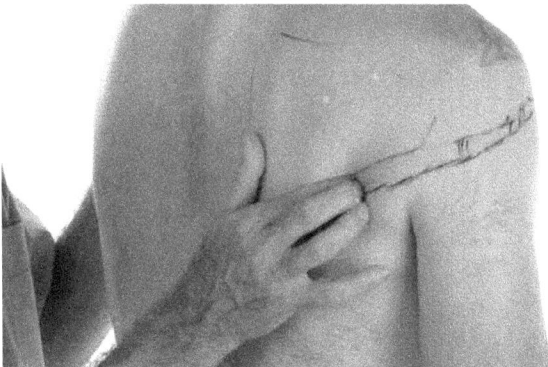

Teres Minor Location

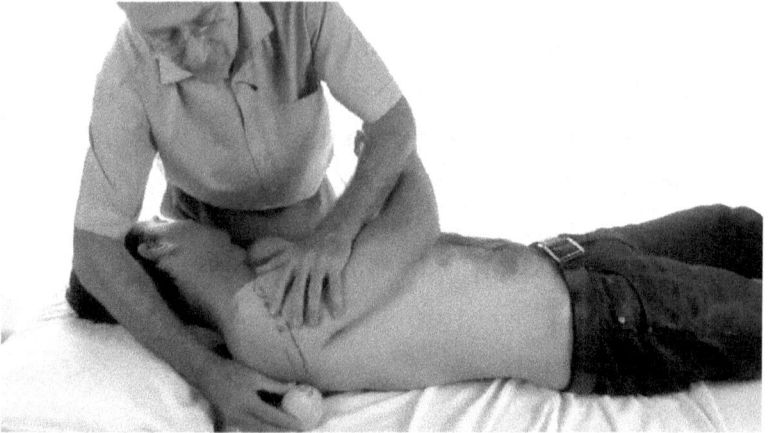

Teres Minor Theracane

Teres Minor Tennis Ball Treatment

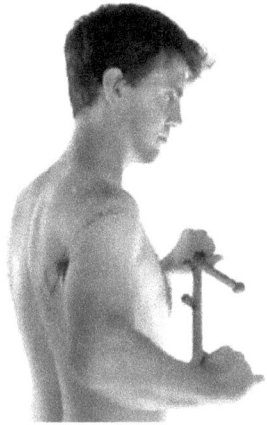

You can, then, use cold therapy by simply running a cold pack over the muscle, starting with the pack near the scapula and sweeping it across the skin over the shoulder joint and down the arm. Do about 2 to 3 sweeps.

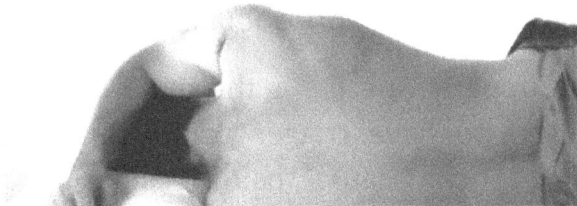

Once you've completed this, it's time to stretch the teres minor. Lay on your side and bring your arm over top of your head. Bend your elbow so your arm is toward the back of your head, and use neuromuscular breathing techniques to deepen the stretch.

Teres Minor Stretch

Afterwards, apply heat for 5 to 10 minutes, then stretch again.

The Trapezius Muscle

The trapezius muscle is a triangle-shaped muscle with 3 parts, the upper, middle, and lower portions. This muscle helps stabilize and move the scapula, including helping to shrug your shoulders.

The upper trapezius is the most common muscle to have trigger points. Trapezius triggers can cause pain locally in the shoulder and up into the base of your skull and forward into your temple.

It's also the major posture muscle of the shoulder girdle and can cause tension headaches. Usually, there are 2 main triggers in the upper trapezius, as pictured.

So, let's take a closer look at how you can

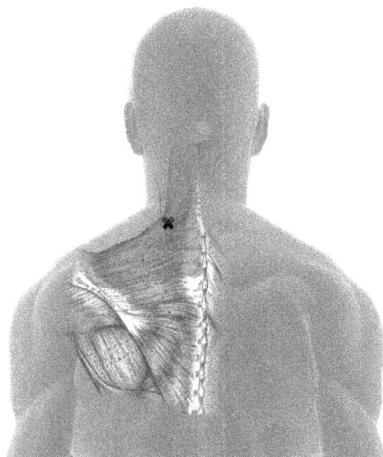

treat this muscle's trigger points and eliminate your pain.

Trapezius Trigger Points #1

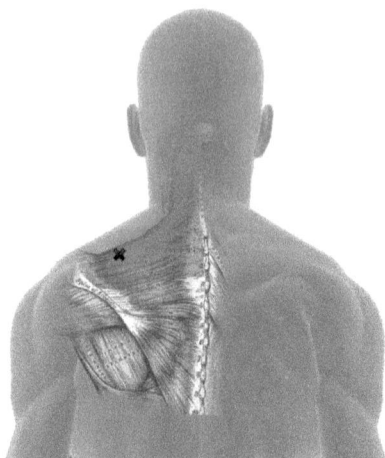

Trapezius Trigger Points #2

Treating Trapezius Trigger Points

Use the fingers of your opposite hand or a theracane to locate your trigger points and apply ischemic pressure principles. Afterwards, you can stretch this muscle.

Upper Trapezius Ischemic Treatment

Upper Trapezius Theracane

To do this, sit or stand up tall. Place your arm behind your back or sit on your hand. Use your other hand to guide your head down, bringing your ear toward your shoulder while keeping your gaze forward. Reach your limit, then use neuromuscular breathing techniques to elongate and relax the muscle even further. Apply heat for 5 to 10 minutes, then stretch again.

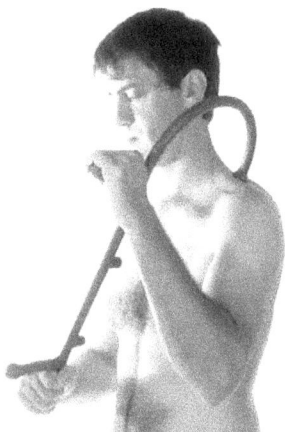

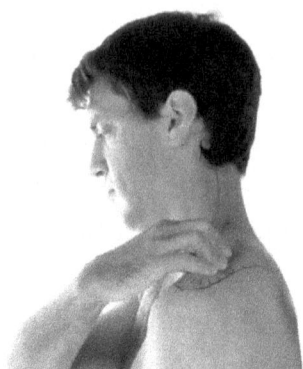

Chapter 4: Chest & Abdomen

Chest & Abdomen Trigger Points

Chronic abdominal pain is a surprisingly common condition. It's very common in children, with about 40% of kids experiencing an episode of chronic abdominal pain. In contrast, about 25% of adults experience significant abdominal pain.

Undeniably, there are many causes of abdominal pain. In most cases, the pain arises from the organs in the abdomen, such as the liver, stomach, or kidneys. However, these are often associated with trigger points in the abdominal wall. Sometimes, these triggers are the primary causes. Yet, most often, they are the secondary cause of pain. So, let's examine how you can effectively abolish this type of pain and relieve abdominal and chest trigger points.

Choosing the Correct Muscle to Treat

On the next page, you'll see pictures of the pain patterns created by trigger points in the chest & abdomen muscles. This exercise is like picking suspects out of a lineup.

Find the one (or two) pain patterns that most match what you're feeling, and navigate to that muscle in this chapter.

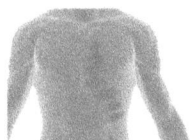
Intercostals

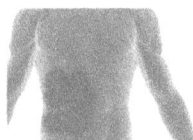
Rectus Abdominus

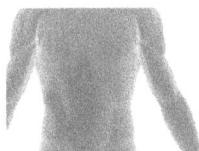
Obliques

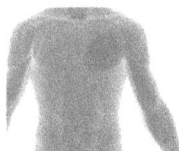
Pectoralis Major

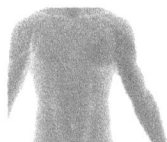
Pectoralis Minor

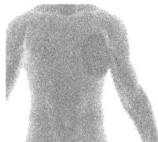
Serratus Anterior

Links to muscles:

Intercostals | Rectus Abdominus & Obliques | Pectorals | Serratus Anterior

The Intercostals

The intercostals are the very small muscles that hold your rib cage together. They are positioned in between the ribs and run all the way around to the back of the body. Essentially, they help raise your ribs up as you breathe in and also help expel air. t's quite hard to find information about trigger points in these muscles. They do exist though, and when they are turned on they can cause sharp localized pain.

Triggers, in this area, are sometimes caused by coughing a lot, such as due to a chest illness or from impact injuries, such as a car crash. The trigger points can be found anywhere within the space between the ribs. So, how can you get rid of them?

Intercostal Trigger Points

Treating Intercostal Trigger Points

Ischemic pressure actually has limited use in this area. For safety reasons, you can only really use a small amount of pressure. However, myofascial release is quite useful here. To perform this, take both of your index fingers and place them on either side of your trigger point.

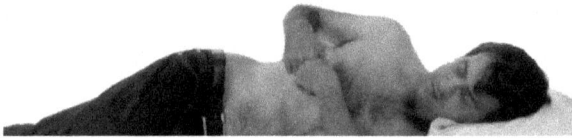

Intercostals Ischemic Treatment

Rest your knuckles together, using them as a lever and pull your fingers apart, stretching the area laterally and medially. This stretches the muscle fibers.

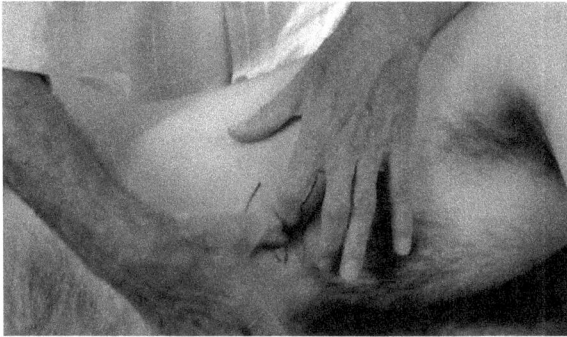

Intercostals Myofascial Release

You can also do this as often as you like and apply heat afterwards for 5 to 10 minutes.

The Rectus Abdominis & Obliques

The obliques are important core stabilizers. They also help twist the torso. The rectus abdominis, on the other hand, is more commonly known as the 'abdominals,' 'abs,' or 'six pack.'

These are the muscles you use when you do crunches or sit ups. Both sets of muscles are used for core strength, stability, and movement.

For trigger points that occur in the rectus abdominis, they can refer pain into your back and tummy. A person can also experience somatic and visceral pain with triggers in this area.

Review the picture below to gain a better understanding of the common trigger points in both of these muscles. Now, let's look at how you can treat these trigger points and feel better.

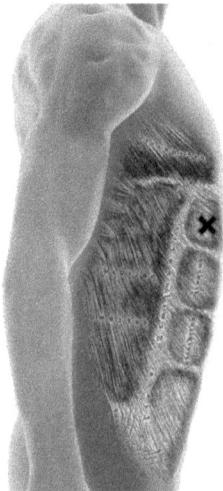

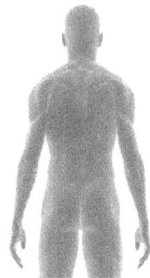

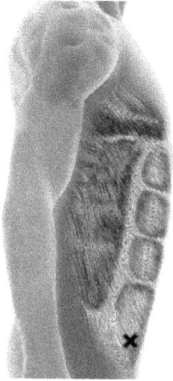

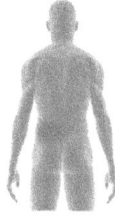

Rectus Abdominus Trigger Points #1

Rectus Abdominus Trigger Points #2

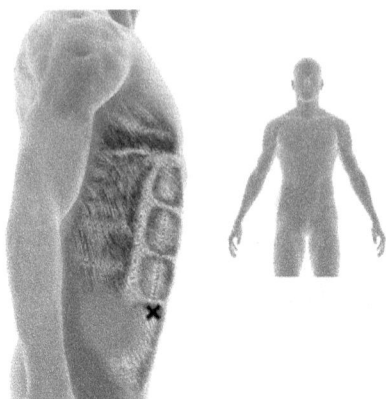

Rectus Abdominus Trigger Points #3

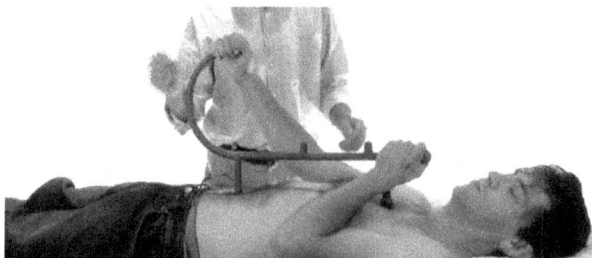

Rectus Abdominus Trigger Points #4

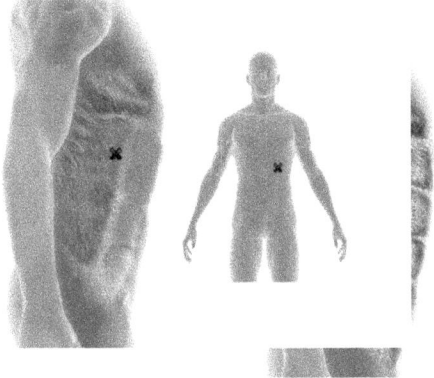

Obliques Trigger Points #1

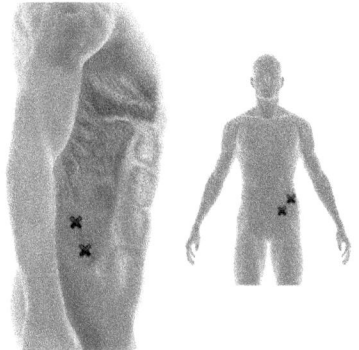

Treating Rectus Abdominis & Oblique Trigger Points

For both the rectus abdominis and obliques, you can use ischemic pressure principles via the use of your fingers or the theracane.

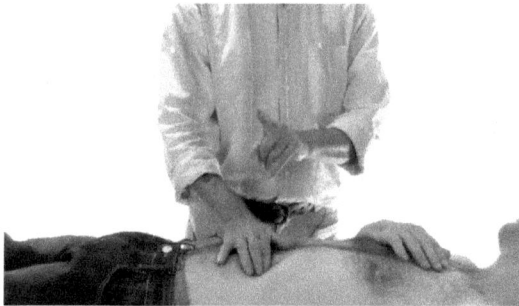

Rectus Abdominus Ischemic Pressure

Rectus Abdominus Theracane

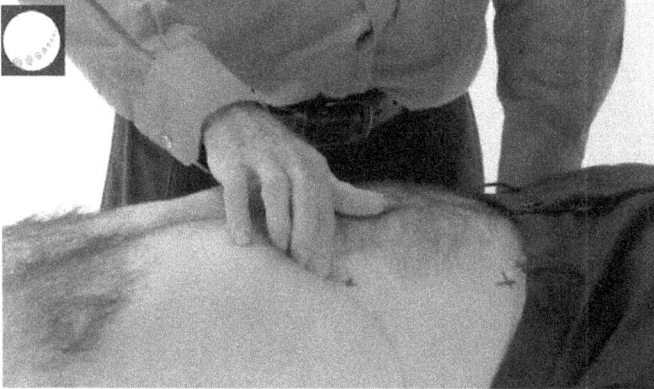

Obliques Ischemic Treatment

Obliques Ischemic Treatment

Afterwards, you can use cold therapy. For the rectus abdominis, this involves starting at the bottom of the muscle and moving the cold pack upwards, performing 2 to 3 sweeps.

For stretching the rectus abdominis, you can lay on your bed, with your feet off the end of the bed, and lean back. As you lean back, breathe in, which should help stretch the abdominal wall.

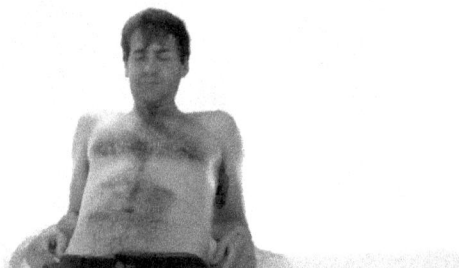

Rectus Abdominus Stretch

For the obliques, you can sweep the cold pack across the abdominals, starting on the outer edge and going toward the midline of the body. Perform 2 to 3 sweeps. For stretching this area, you can perform the same stretch as the rectus abdominis but with an additional twist or slight rotation of the torso.

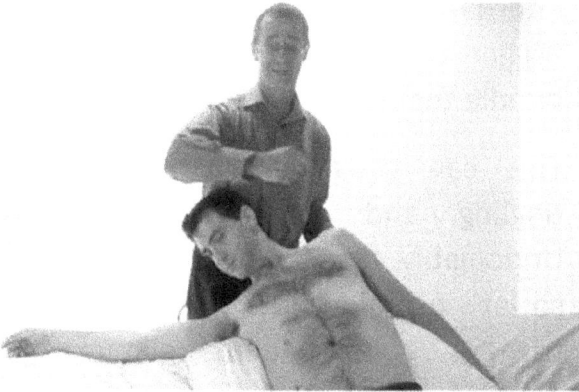

Obliques Stretch

For both stretches, follow the neuromuscular breathing techniques to fully elongate and eliminate those trigger points. Apply heat for 5 to 10 minutes after doing so.

Pectoralis Major and Minor

The pectoralis muscles, often simply called the chest muscles, are located in the upper torso (as illustrated in the picture). The pectoralis major trigger points refer pain locally, into the shoulder and down the arm. When the pectoralis minor, which internally rotates the arm, has active trigger points, it can constrict the nerve bundle that runs into your arm.

This can cause sharp shooting pains, tingling, and numbness in your arm. Undeniably, this can be quite bothersome, so let's examine how you can treat these trigger points and eliminate any discomforts.

Pectoralis Minor Trigger Points

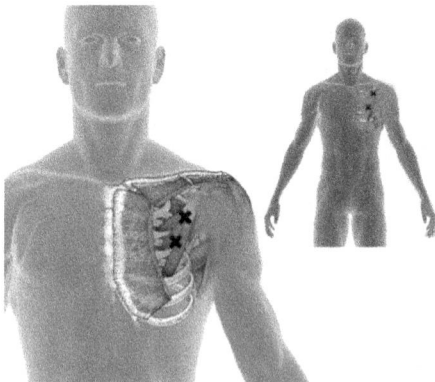

Pectoralis Major Trigger Points #1

Pectoralis Major Trigger Points #2

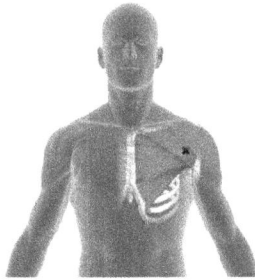

Pectoralis Major Trigger Points #3

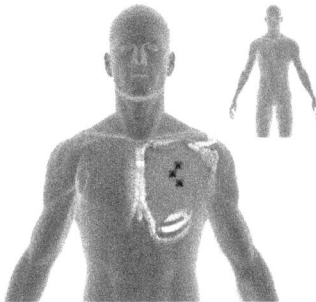

129

Treating Pectoralis Major and Minor Trigger Points

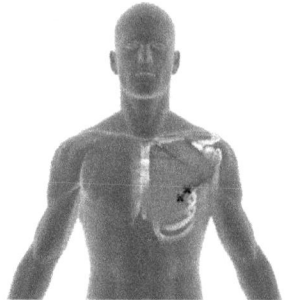

For the pectoralis major and minor, you can use your hand from your opposite side or use the theracane to determine the location of your trigger points. As you press in, you should feel pain. You can then reduce your pressure so that you are just under the pain threshold. From here, you can apply the ischemic pressure principles to deactivate the trigger.

Pectoralis Minor Ischemic Pressure

Pectoralis Minor Theracane

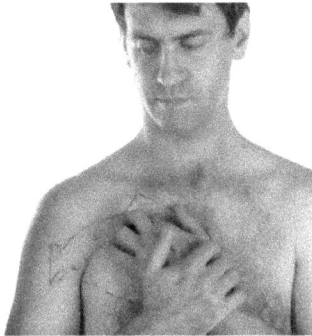

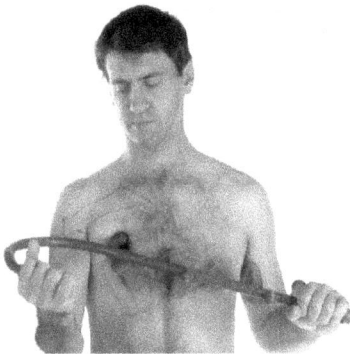

Pectoralis Major Ischemic Pressure

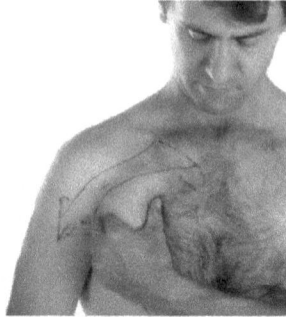

Pectoralis Major Ischemic Pressure

You can use cold on both of these muscles, starting from the midline and sweeping it across to the point of insertion and pain zone. Move the cold pack at a pace of about 2 to 3 centimeters per second and do about 2 to 3 sweeps. This further deactivates the trigger point as it acts as a distraction.

From there, you can stretch these areas. The stretch you perform depends on where your trigger point is located. Although, it can help to stretch the entire area to truly eliminate those trigger points and relieve tightness. For stretching the chest, stand tall in a door frame. Bend your elbows and place your forearms on the door frame so that your elbows are above shoulder height.

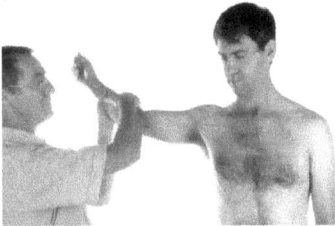

Pectoralis Minor Stretch

Pectoralis Major Stretch

Step in until you feel a stretch. This targets the lower portion of the chest muscles. For stretching the middle portion, lower your elbows so that they are in line with your shoulders and repeat. For the higher portion of the muscles, lower your forearms and elbows so that they are below your shoulder and chest level.

You can then follow this up with heat for 5 to 10 minutes, and even repeat the stretch afterwards.

The Serratus Anterior Muscle

The serratus anterior muscle runs along the scapula to the ribs. This muscle helps stabilize and protract the scapula. The trigger point in this muscle is often found in the middle, as illustrated in the picture.

When trigger points occur here, they can reduce normal movement of the ribs and restrict breathing. It might feel as though a tight band is around your chest. Thus, eliminating these triggers can provide a ton of relief.

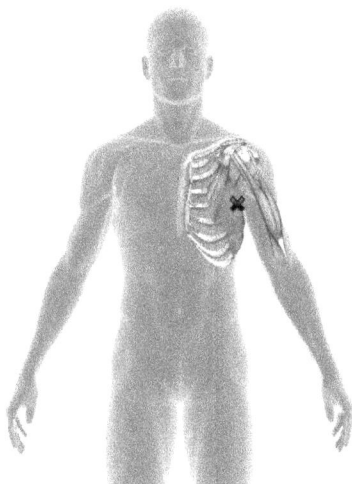

Serratus Anterior Trigger Points

Serratus Posterior Trigger Points

Treating Serratus Anterior Trigger Points

Use your opposite hand to press into the trigger point. Use enough pressure to

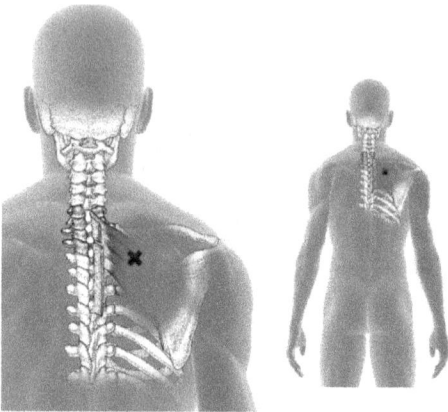

cause pain, then reduce it so that you are just above the pain threshold. Continue to follow ischemic principles to deactivate the trigger point. You can also use the theracane here if you so choose.

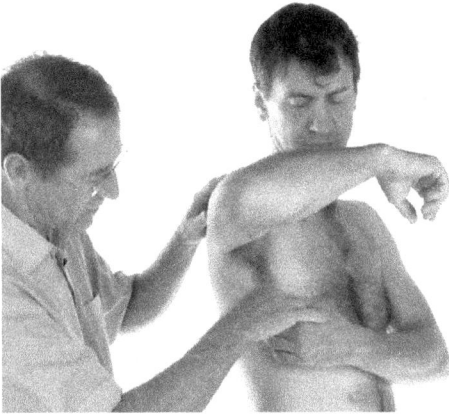

Serratus Anterior Ischemic Pressure

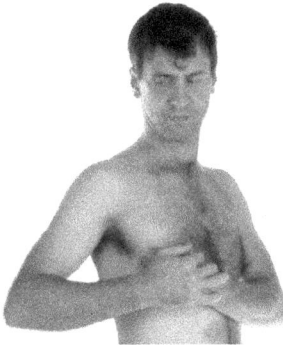

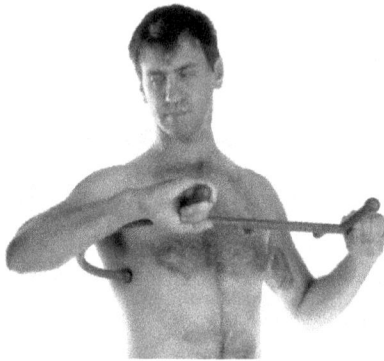

Serratus Anterior Ischemic Pressure

Serratus Anterior Theracane

Afterwards, use cold therapy, sweeping a cold pack from the ribs backwards toward the origin at the spatula. You may need your partner or a friend to help you do this. Have them perform 2 to 3 sweeps.

Following this, you can stretch the muscle. This helps relieve tightness and prevents the trigger point from being reactivated. To do this, rest your hand on your hip with your elbow bent backwards and your scapula intending backwards.

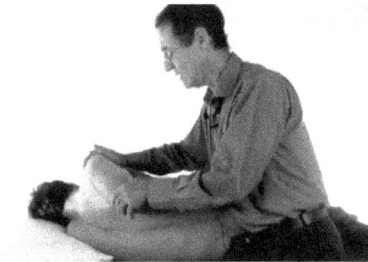

Serratus Anterior Stretch

Hold here, using neuromuscular breathing techniques to deepen the stretch. Once completed, apply heat for 5 to 10 minutes. You should notice redness afterwards which indicates increased blood flow to the area.

Chapter 5: Arm & Hand

Arm & Hand Trigger Points

About 16% of the general population complains about pain in the hands. This isn't surprising since the hands perform various fine motor tasks throughout a person's day. In fact, many reported hand pain cases are related to recurring tasks, such as typing or using a computer mouse.

Big movements with the hands arise from the muscles in the forearms, and almost everybody will have trigger points in their dominant hand at some point, especially around the forearm. In individuals with arthritis, trigger points can be a secondary cause of pain.

Yet, in many other instances, trigger points in the hands and forearms are the primary cause of pain. So, let's take a look at the muscles of the forearm and hand and uncover how you can reduce and potentially eliminate your trigger points and pain.

Choosing the Correct Muscle to Treat

On the next page, you'll see pictures of the pain patterns created by trigger points in the arm & hand muscles. This exercise is like picking suspects out of a lineup.

Find the one (or two) pain patterns that most match what you're feeling, and navigate to that muscle in this chapter.

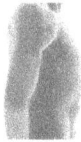

Biceps

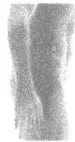

Brachioradialis

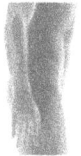

Forearm Extensors

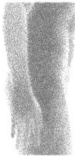

Hand Intrinsics

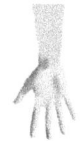

Thenar Emminence

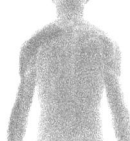

Triceps

Links to muscles:

The Biceps Muscle

The biceps is a 'workhorse' muscle that goes across 2 joints – your shoulder and elbow joint. This muscle is unusual because it has a tendon that runs through a joint.

The biceps stabilize the shoulder joint and are required for heavy lifting. This muscle has two heads, the short head and long head. When this muscle contracts, it flexes the shoulder and elbow.

Triggers are frequently set off from heavy lifting requiring flexion (bending) of the elbow. This muscle usually has two triggers in the center and fattest part of the muscle, one on the long head and one on the short head.

These triggers often refer pain up into your shoulder and then down into your elbow – they don't actually refer pain locally. So, how can you tackle these triggers?

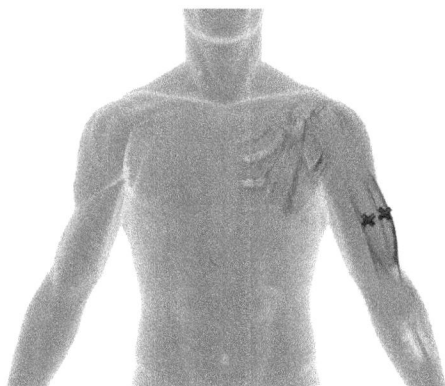

Biceps Trigger Points

Treating Bicep Trigger Points

Take the whole bicep muscle in your hand and squeeze it until you find a trigger point. Using your finger, apply ischemic principles until the trigger point is turned off. If you have a particularly big muscle, you may need to use your fist to apply this pressure.

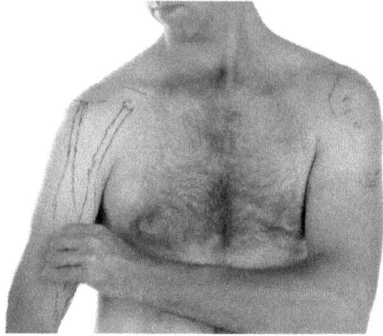

Biceps Ischemic Treatment

Afterwards, you can use cold therapy to further turn off that trigger point. If your pain is primarily in front of your shoulder, begin a sweeping movement with the cold pack near the elbow, moving up at a pace of 2 to 3 centimeters per second. Perform about 2 to 3 sweeps.

From there, you can stretch the muscle. Do this by finding a door frame. Place your arm straight behind you with your palm facing backwards on the door frame.

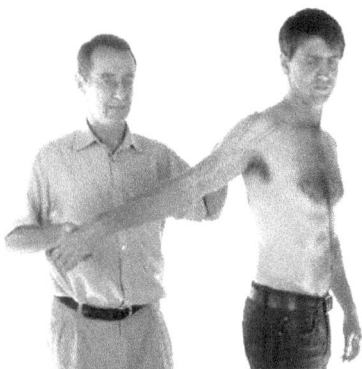

Biceps Stretch #1

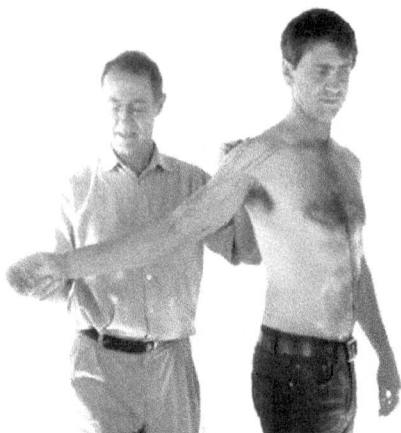

Biceps Stretch #2

Turn your body away and you should feel a gentle stretch through the bicep muscle.

Use neuromuscular principles and breathing to reset the range of motion and to give the muscle a thorough stretch and release.

The Brachioradialis Muscle

The brachioradialis muscle, as illustrated below, has a long origin where it inserts into the lower part of the humerus. It, then, runs over the elbow joint and attaches to the styloid process of the radius bone.

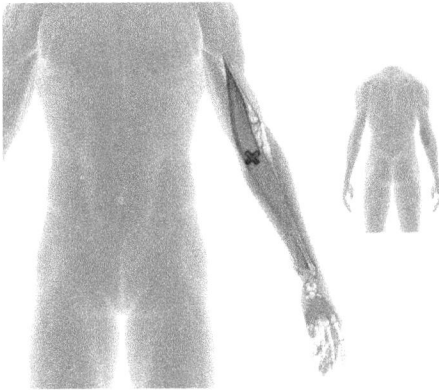

The main function of this muscle is to flex the elbow, and trigger points commonly occur in the largest part of the bellow of this muscle, as pictured. These trigger points can cause pain in two areas; the lateral epicondyle of the elbow (mimicking tennis elbow) and the area between the thumb and the index finger. So, let's explore how you can treat this muscle and its trigger points.

Treating Brachioradialis Trigger Points

Using your opposite hand squeeze the brachioradialis muscle in between your thumb and index fingers. Squeeze until you find a trigger point. Alternatively, you can move your index finger back and forth along the belly of the muscle until you find

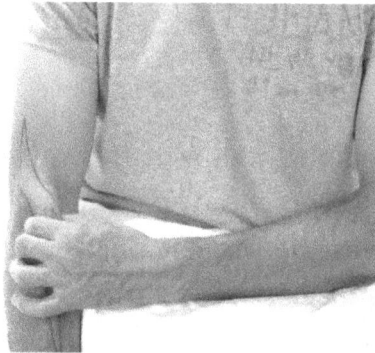

the trigger, then press in and follow ischemic pressure principles. You can also use the theracane to treat these arm trigger points, if you so choose.

Brachioradialis Ischemic Pressure

Brachioradialis Theracane

Once you've directly treated the trigger, use a cold pack to further distract and reduce the trigger point. If the trigger point is referring pain upwards, start at the end of the muscle closest to your hand and sweep the ice pack up. Perform 2 to 3 sweeps, then stretch.

For stretching the brachioradialis, straighten your arm in front of you. Drop the wrist down with your palm facing toward you and rotate your wrist slightly away from the midline of the body using your opposite hand.

Brachioradialis Stretch

Once you've reached your limit, follow the neuromuscular breathing techniques to relax and stretch the muscle further.

The Forearm Extensors

These muscles extend (lift up) the hand at the wrist and straighten the fingers out. The forearm extensors consist of the extensor carpi ulnaris, the extensor carpi radialis brevis, the extensor carpi radialis longus, and extensor digitorum.

The carpi radialis brevis and longus extend the wrist and deviate the wrist toward the thumb side, contracting together.

The extensor carpi ulnaris dorsi flexes the wrist, pulling the wrist slightly up and deviating it to the ulnar side. The extensor carpi ulnaris' primary function is actually to hold your hand up so you can grip. Meanwhile, the extensor digitorum's main function is to extend the fingers.

In these muscles, triggers are caused by recurrent use of these muscles, such as when playing the keyboard or when playing certain instruments. Pain is frequently felt in the wrist, hand, and fingers.

There is also often weakness and stiffness in your grip and a loss of rapid movements in the fingers. So, let's find out how you can reduce these symptoms and eliminate

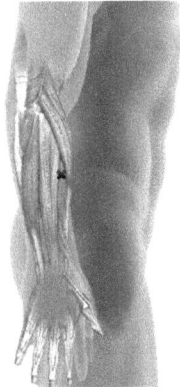

your trigger points.

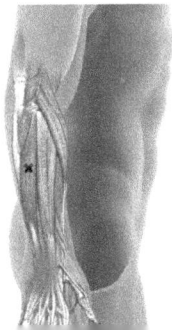

Forearm Extensor Trigger Points #1

Forearm Extensor Trigger Points #2

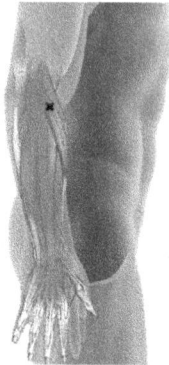

Forearm Extensor Trigger Points #3

Treating Forearm Extensor Trigger Points

Place your finger on the muscle you suspect is the problem. Using the pictures below, you can determine which muscle may be causing you pain.

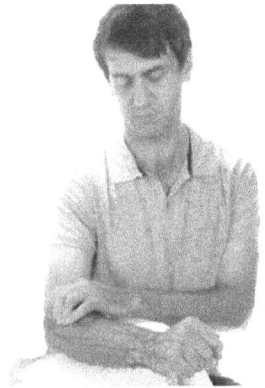

Forearm Extensor Ischemic Treatment

Go back and forth with your finger until you find a tight band, then go along until you find the tender point. From there, follow the ischemic pressure principles to deactivate the trigger point. Afterwards, place heat on for about 5 to 10 minutes, then stretch the muscle.

For the ischemic pressure phase, you can also choose to use a theracane. For stretching the extensor carpi radialis long, place your opposite hand on the wrist and

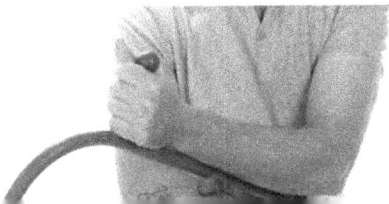

pull the hand down and slightly away from the midline of the body.

Forearm Extensor Theracane

For the extensor carpi radialis brevis, use your opposite hand to pull your wrist straight down, with your palm facing toward you. For stretching the extensor carpi ulnaris, use your opposite hand to pull the hand down, with the palm toward you again, and also slightly inward, toward the midline of the body.

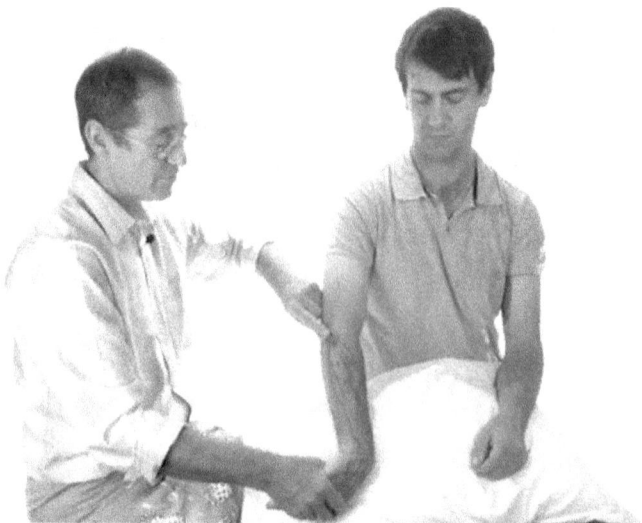

Forearm Extensor Stretch

To stretch the extensor digitorum, curl your fingers into a fist, place your opposite hand over your finger and curl the hand down. Afterwards, you can apply heat for

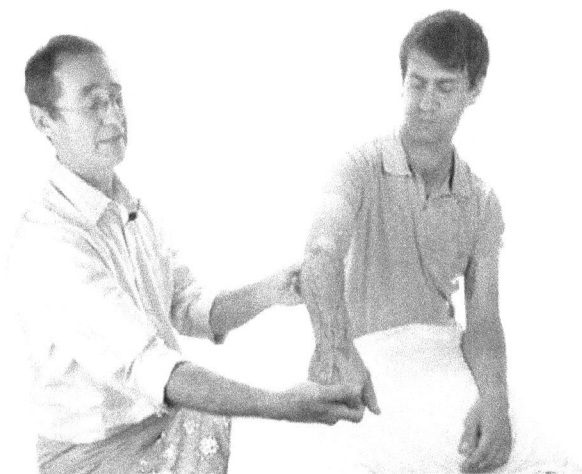

5 to 10 minutes.

Forearm Extensor Stretch

For further distraction and elimination of the trigger point, you can use a cold pack, right out of the freezer, and sweep it over the trigger points and pain zone by starting at the origin of the muscle. Sweep the cold pack across at a 2 to 3 centimetres per second pace. Do this 2 to 3 times.

The Intrinsics of the Hand

The intrinsics of the hand move the fingers toward and away from the midline of the hand. They are particularly useful for fine manipulation of objects. Yet, this means that trigger points in this area are often caused by repetitive and/or forceful pincer grips.

With trigger points in the intrinsics of the hand, you'll frequently have pain and stiffness in the fingers and awkwardness with fine motor movements. The pain is usually locally located, right at the trigger point, but it may also include pain running down the finger or thumb. So, let's examine how you can address these trigger points.

Intrinsics of Hand #1

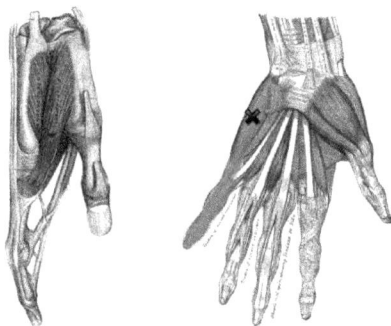

Intrinsics of Hand #2

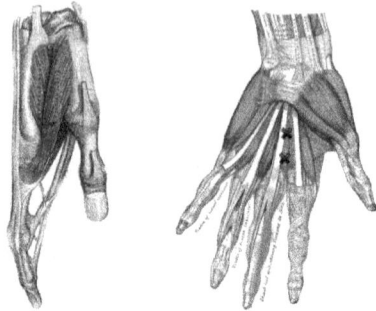

Intrinsics of Hand #3

Treating Intrinsics of the Hand Trigger Points

With these small muscles, it's really difficult to use pressure outside, with the exception of the area between the thumb and index fingers, which is actually a common trigger and acupuncture point, and the area on the outside of the hand near the pinky finger.

You can use ischemic pressure principles to address these triggers and deactivate them. After treatment, apply heat for 5 to 10 minutes, then perform a stretch.

Hand Intrinsics Ischemic Pressure

To stretch the intrinsics of the hand, put your fingers together, with each finger touching the same finger of the opposite hand, then spread your fingers and thumbs out, pushing slightly together without your wrists touching.

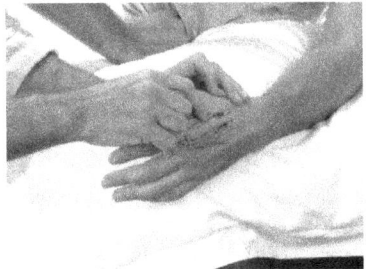

Hand Intrinsics Stretch

159

You can use neuromuscular breathing techniques to deepen the stretch further, then apply heat again afterwards.

The Thenar Eminence Muscles

The thenar eminence muscles pull the thumb inwards and also rotate it to meet the tips of the fingers. These muscles are crucial for a pincer grip and to be able to manipulate objects.

The two muscles pictured that make up the thenar eminence include the adductor pollicis (which pulls the thumb toward the midline of the hand) and the opponens pollicis (which brings the tip of the thumb into contact with the other fingers).

Trigger points arise from strong prolonged pincer grip, such as with weeding, sewing, and writing. Individuals often experience pain in the wrist and thumb (as illustrated) with stiffness and interference with fine motor skills of the hand. Now, let's take a look at how to treat the thenar eminence trigger points.

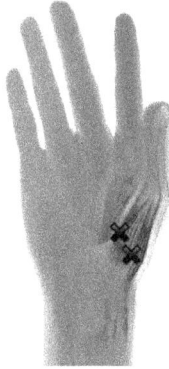

Thenar Eminence Trigger Points

Treating Thenar Eminence Trigger Points

Feel along the muscles until you find a tight band, then continue until you find a painful point. Extending the thumb can actually make it easier to locate triggers in this area. Once you find a trigger, support your index finger with your middle finger and use ischemic pressure principles to deactivate the trigger point.

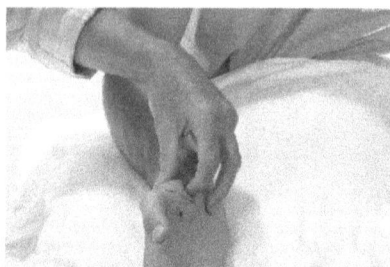

Thenar Emminence Ischemic Treatment

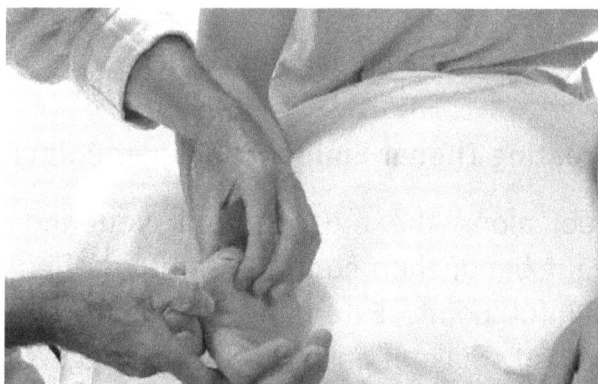

Thenar Emminence Ischemic Treatment

Using a cold pack, start at the origin of the muscle (closer to the wrist) and run up and across the pain zone. Perform 2 to 3 sweeps, then stretch.

From here, you'll want to stretch the problematic muscle. For stretching the adductor, grab your thumb with your opposite hand and gently pull it away from your fingers.

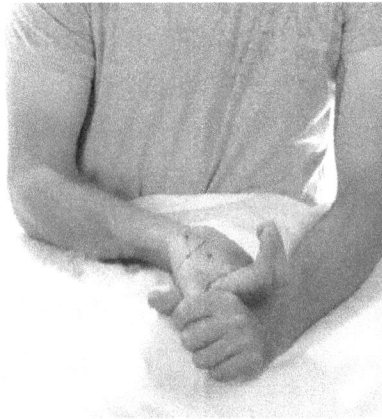

Thenar Emminence Stretch

For your opponens pollicis, gently pull your thumb back. For both stretches, you can use the neuromuscular breathing techniques to achieve a greater range of motion.

The Triceps Muscle

The triceps muscle works closely with your latissimus dorsi muscle. It's used extensively when swimming, performing push-ups, and for various other powerful arm movements. Basically, any movement that straightens the arm involves the triceps.

Trigger points in the triceps frequently cause pain in the back of the arm. The most common trigger points occur in the

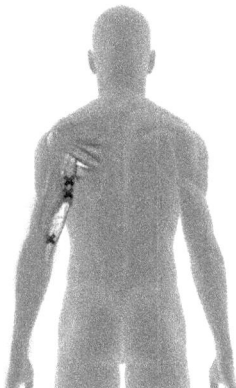

third head of this muscle, as pictured, and radiate pain to the back of the shoulder joint and elbow, sometimes mimicking tennis elbow. So, let's find out how to treat these triggers!

Triceps Trigger Points #1

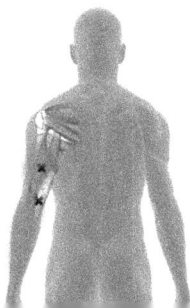

Treating Tricep Trigger Points

Lift your affected arm slightly up so you have enough room to place your hand underneath and be able to dig into the triceps with your fingers. Feel for the trigger point. You can pinch your muscles to do this, if needed. Once you find that

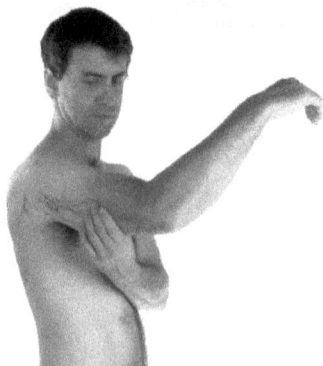

tender spot, apply ischemic pressure principles.

Triceps Ischemic Treatment

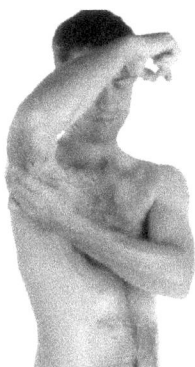

Triceps Ischemic Treatment

Afterwards, use a cold pack to distract the trigger point and deactivate it even further. Start at the insertion (shoulder) and sweep the pack over the pain zone and triggers. Do about 2 to 3 sweeps at a pace of about 2 to 3 centimeters per second.

Then, you can stretch the triceps. Do this by lifting your arm straight up, bending your elbow, and allowing your hand to fall behind your head. You can then use your

opposite hand to gently pull the elbow
back.

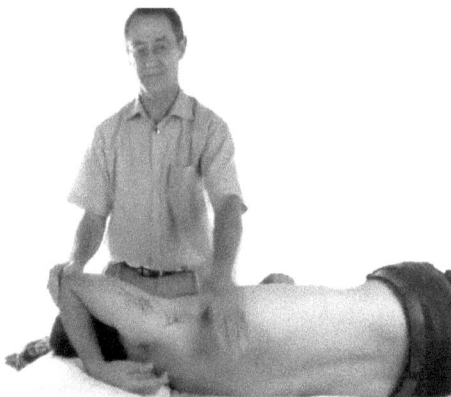

Triceps Stretch

Once you've reached your limit, you can
use the neuromuscular breathing
technique, described earlier in this book,
to fully stretch and relax the muscle, then
apply heat for 5 to 10 minutes.

Chapter 6: Lower Back & Pelvis

Lower Back, Pelvis & Buttocks Trigger Points

The World Health Organization (WHO) reported that 44% of adults have experienced pain in the lower back in the last month. Maybe you've experienced low back pain or you know someone that has. Either way, this pain can be incredibly disruptive and debilitating.

When trigger points are addressed and treated in these areas, the pain often goes away. Undeniably, the back is a very complex structure with various muscles helping balance and move the torso each day.

The buttocks muscles are also used everyday, helping propel your body forward, helping you stand from a sitting position, and more. So, let's dive into this part of the body a little further and learn how to reduce trigger points in the lower back, pelvis, and buttocks.

Choosing the Correct Muscle to Treat

On the next page, you'll see pictures of the pain patterns created by trigger points in the lower back and buttock muscles. This exercise is like picking suspects out of a lineup.

Find the one (or two) pain patterns that most match what you're feeling, and

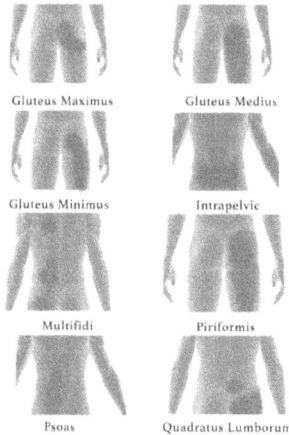

Gluteus Maximus Gluteus Medius

Gluteus Minimus Intrapelvic

Multifidi Piriformis

Psoas Quadratus Lumborum

navigate to that muscle in this chapter.

Muscle Links:

The Gluteus Maximus

The gluteus maximus is a big power muscle in the buttocks. This muscle extends and laterally rotates the hip joint, which means we use it every single day for walking, running, and standing. This muscle further has the advantage of being superficial compared to the other glute muscles, making trigger points in this area relatively easy to access.

There are 3 main trigger points, as illustrated. Pain is often felt locally and slightly higher up from the muscle, so let's look at how you can reduce this pain.

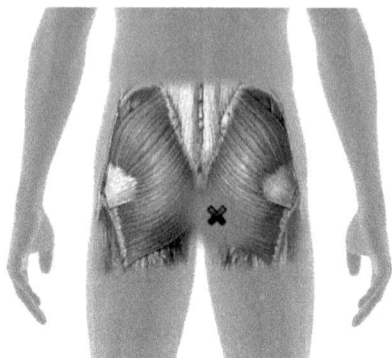

Gluteus Maximus Trigger Points #1

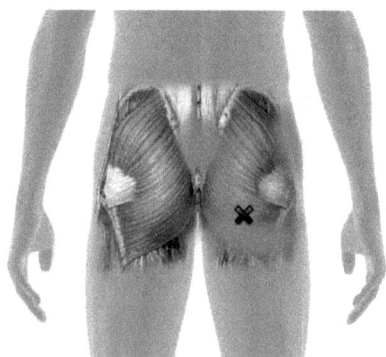

Gluteus Maximus Trigger Points #2

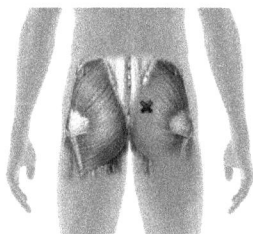

Gluteus Maximus Trigger Points #3

Treating Gluteus Maximus Trigger Points

Lying down or on your side, use your hand to pinch the muscle and find the trigger point. Alternatively, you can use a theracane or lacrosse ball. Push hard enough until you feel pain, then back off,

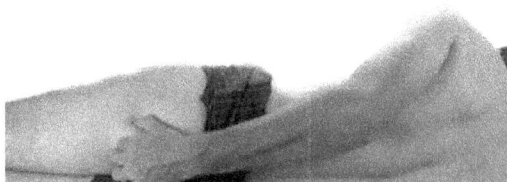

and follow the ischemic pressure principles to deactivate the trigger point.

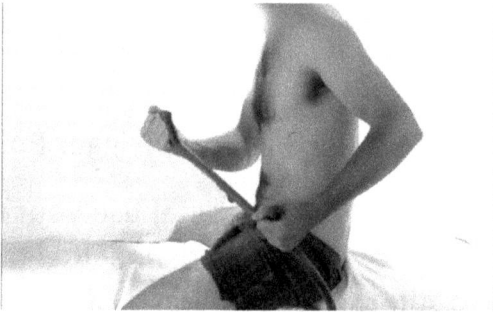

Gluteus Maximus Ischemic Treatment

Gluteus Maximus Theracane

For cold therapy and further deactivation of the trigger, grab an ice pack from your freezer and sweep the cold from the top of the glute and down over the pain zone and triggers. You may need a friend or partner to help you do this.

Afterwards, you can stretch the gluteus maximus. Because the muscle is an extensor, you want to perform the opposite movement by bending the leg and pulling the knee close into the chest. This is easier to do lying on your side or back. Once you reach your limit, use neuromuscular breathing techniques to elongate and fully stretch the muscle.

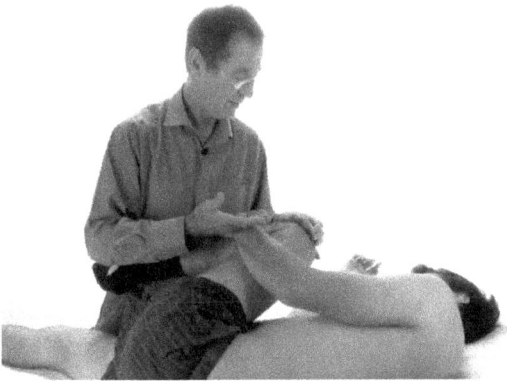

Gluteus Maximus Stretch

Once you perform the stretch, apply heat for 5 to 10 minutes. After this, you can perform another stretch to ensure a full release of that shortened muscle.

The Gluteus Minimus and Medius

The two muscles, the gluteus minimus and gluteus medius, are located underneath the gluteus maximus. The gluteus minimus muscle can mimic the pain of sciatica – which means pain may run right down your leg. Meanwhile, the gluteus medius often refers pain locally, as illustrated in the picture.

The gluteus minimus and medius act in synergy with one another, helping to abduct and internally rotate the thigh. For trigger points and referred pain in these muscles, view the picture below. Now, let's explore how you can eliminate these painful and tender spots.

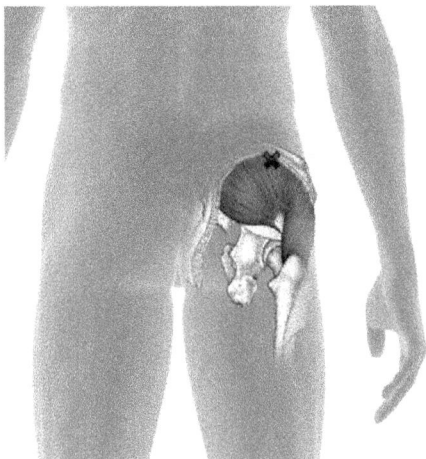

Gluteus Medius Trigger Points #1

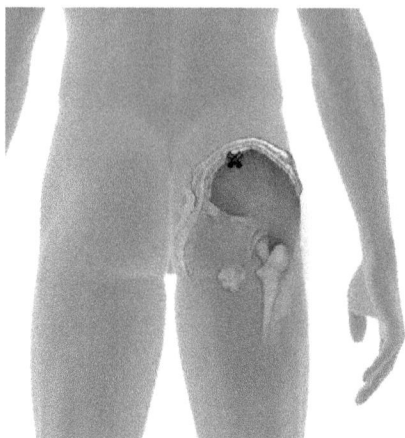

Gluteus Medius Trigger #2

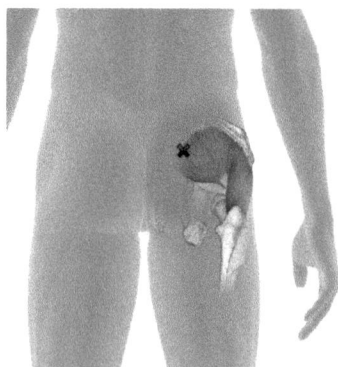

Gluteus Medius Trigger Points #3

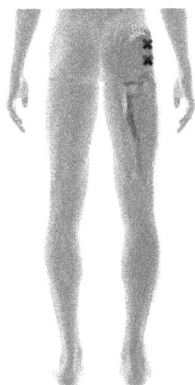

Gluteus Minimus Trigger Points #1

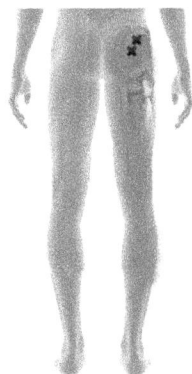

Gluteus Minimus Trigger Points #2

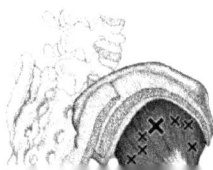

Gluteus Minimus Trigger Points #3

Treating Gluteus Minimus and Medius Trigger Points

Find the trigger points by pressing into the muscle with the use of your thumb, theracane, or lacrosse ball. If you're using your thumb, you can also use your other hand to help apply pressure. Once you find a tight band, go along the band until you

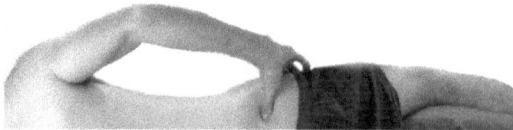

find that really painful spot. Once there, apply ischemic pressure principles.

Gluteus Minimus Ischemic Treatment

Gluteus Minimus Theracane

For cold therapy and to distract the trigger, use an ice pack and start at the origin, going toward the insertion and along the pain zones, in a gentle sweep. Perform about 2 to 3 sweeps. If pain refers down, start at the top and go down. If the pain refers up, start down and move up.

Afterwards, you can stretch the muscle to relieve tension and tightness. Lie on your side on a bed, and bring your leg straight forward off the bed so it hangs. This stretch targets the triggers further in the back.

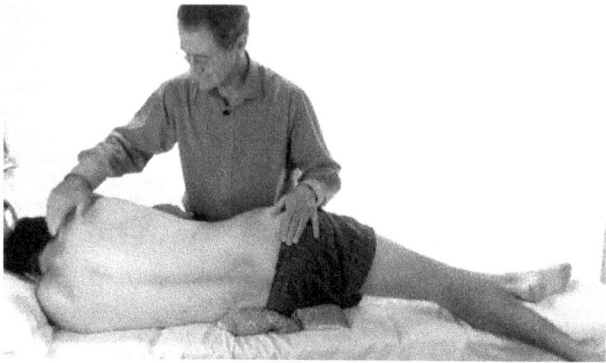

Gluteus Minimus Stretch

If the triggers are closer to the front of the muscle, lie on your side and move your leg back and hang it off the bed behind you. You can then apply heat for 5 to 10 minutes, before stretching again.

The Intra Pelvic Muscles

When triggers in these muscles cause problems, it can make life very difficult. And unfortunately, they can only be reached by internal examination by a medical professional. Triggers are common causes of pain and dysfunction in these muscles. They are also very deep, as shown in the picture.

These muscles are incredibly important as they cover the inside of the pelvic bones and essentially keep your insides and organs from falling out.

In women, trigger points in this area are often diagnosed as chronic pelvic pain or even endometriosis. In contrast, other conditions, like endometriosis, can cause trigger points to occur in these areas.

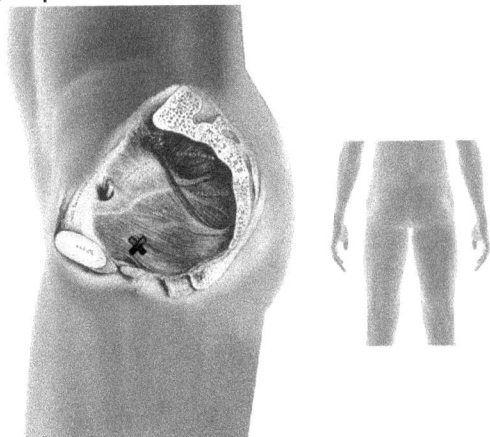

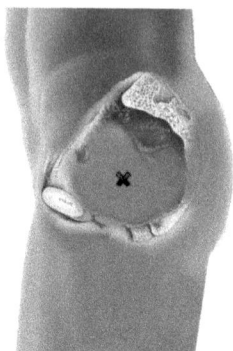

Intrapelvic Trigger Points #1

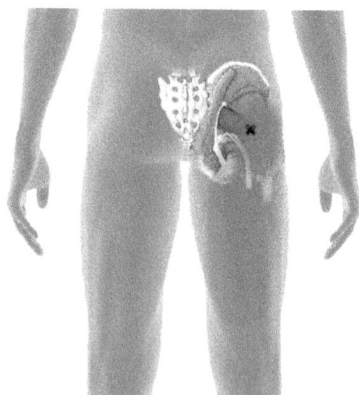